Biomedical Aspects
of IUDs

Advances in Reproductive Health Care

Series Editor: **E.S.E. Hafez**

*Advances in
Reproductive Health Care*

Biomedical Aspects
of IUDs

Editors

H. Hasson, E.S.E. Hafez
and W.A. van Os

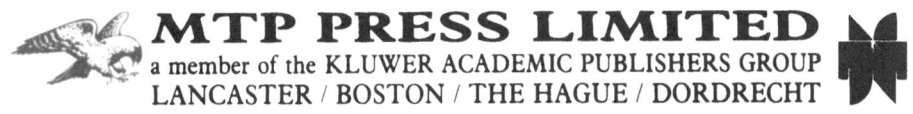

MTP PRESS LIMITED
a member of the KLUWER ACADEMIC PUBLISHERS GROUP
LANCASTER / BOSTON / THE HAGUE / DORDRECHT

Published in the UK and Europe by
MTP Press Limited
Falcon House
Lancaster, England

British Library Cataloguing in Publication Data

Biomedical aspects of IUDs.—(Advances in
reproductive health care)
1. Intrauterine contraceptives
I. Hasson, H.M.   II. Hafez, E.S.E.
III. Os, W.A.A. van   IV. Series
613.9'435   RG137.3

Published in the USA by
MTP Press
A division of Kluwer Boston Inc
190 Old Derby Street
Hingham, MA 02043, USA

Library of Congress Cataloging in Publication Data

Main entry under title:

Biomedical aspects of IUDs.

(Advances in reproductive health care)
Based on presentations made at the Reproductive
Health Care International Symposium, held in Kaanapali,
Hawaii, in Oct. 1982
Includes bibliographies and index.
1. Intrauterine contraceptives—Congresses.
I. Hasson, H. II. Hafez, E. S. E. (Elsayed Saad
Eldin), 1922-   . IV. Reproductive Health Care
International Symposium (1982: Kaanapali, Hawaii)
V. Title: Biomedical aspects of I.U.D.s. VI. Series.
[DNLM: 1. Intrauterine Devices—congresses.
WP 640 B615 1982]
RG137.3.B56 1984   613.9'435   84-23403
ISBN-13: 978-94-010-8668-4   e-ISBN-13: 978-94-009-4896-9
DOI: 10.1007/978-94-009-4896-9

Contents

CONTENTS

List of Contributors

L. ANDOLSEK
Department of Obstetrics and Gynecology, University Medical Centre Ljubljana, Slajmerjeva 3, 61000 Ljubljana, Yugoslavia

R. AZNAR
Jefatura de Servicios de Planificación Familiar, Instituto Mexicano del Seguro Social, Mexico DF, Mexico

G. BERNASCHEK
II Universitäts-Frauenklinik Spitalgasse 23, 1090 Vienna, Austria

H. DERSHIN
Grant Hospital of Chicago, 550 W. Webster Ave., Chicago, Illinois 60614, USA

M. ELSTEIN
Department of Obstetrics & Gynaecology, University Hospitals of South Manchester, West Didsbury, Manchester M20 8LR, United Kingdom

M. GONZALEZ-DIDDI
Jefatura de Servicios de Planificación Familiar, Instituto Mexicano del Seguro Social, Mexico DF, Mexico

M. GUBINA
Institute of Microbiology, University Edvard Kardelj, Zaloška Cesta 2, 61000 Ljubljana, Yugoslavia

H.M. HASSON
Department of Obstetrics and Gynecology, Rush Medical College and Grant Hospital of Chicago, 550 W. Webster Ave., Chicago, Illinois 60614, USA

H. HREN-VENCELJ
Institute of Microbiology, University Edvard Kardelj, Zaloška Cesta 2, 61000 Ljubljana, Yugoslavia

U.J. KOCH
Bismarckstr 67, D-1000, Berlin-39, Federal Republic of Germany

M. KOZUH-NOVAK
Department of Obstetrics and Gynecology, University Centre Ljubljana, Slajmerjeva 3, 61000 Ljubljana, Yugoslavia

B. KRALJ
Department of Obstetrics and Gynecology, University Centre Ljubljana, Slajmerjeva 3, 61000 Ljubljana, Yugoslavia

S. LEVI
Ultrasound Clinic, Department of Gynecology and Obstetrics, University Hospital Brugmann, 1020 Brussels, Belgium

M. LOZANO
Jefatura de Servicios de Planificación Familiar, Instituto Mexicano del Seguro Social, Mexico DF, Mexico

K.S. LUDWIG
Anatomisches Institut der Universität, Pestalozzistr 20, 4056 Basel, Switzerland

M. MALL-HAEFELI
Sozialmedizinischer Dienst der Universitäts-Frauenklinik, 4056 Basel, Switzerland

P.K. MEHROTRA
Division of Endocrinology, Central Drug Research Institute, Chattar Manzil POB.173, Lucknow 226001, India

vii

LIST OF CONTRIBUTORS

I.D. NUTTALL
Department of Obstetrics and Gynaecology, University Hospitals of South Manchester, West Didsbury, Manchester M20 8LR, United Kingdom

L. REYNOSO
Jefatura de Servicios de Planificación Familiar, Instituto Mexicano del Seguro Social, Mexico DF, Mexico

B.W. SIMCOCK
Family Planning Clinic, Department of Obstetrics and Gynecology, Westmead Hospital, Westmead, NSW 2145, Australia

R. SPERNOL
II Universitäts-Frauenklinik, Spitalgasse 23, 1090 Vienna, Austria

U.M. SPORNITZ
Anatomisches Institut der Universität, Pestalozzistr 20, 4056 Basel, Switzerland

K. SRIVASTAVA
Division of Endocrinology, Central Drug Research Institute, Chattar Manzil POB 173, Lucknow 226001, India

G. ZAMORA
Jefatura de Servicios de Planificación Familiar, Instituto Mexicano del Seguro Social, Mexico DF, Mexico

Preface

This volume contains a collection of papers based on presentations made at the Reproductive Health Care International Symposium held in Maui, Hawaii, USA, October 1982. The papers evaluate biologic interactions between intrauterine contraceptive devices and the host, examine the risks associated with the use of these devices and describe aspects of technical progress in the field. The contributing authors bring their knowledge and expertise from four corners of the world to the readers.

The editors wish to express their appreciation to the authors for their valuable contributions, to Carolyn K. Osborn for helpful assistance in editing the manuscripts and to MTP Press for accurate preparation and fine presentation of the material.

It is hoped that this volume will serve to expand knowledge and generate further interest among its readers in the dynamic and fascinating field of intrauterine contraception.

April, 1984
Chicago, Illinois, USA

H.M. Hasson, MD

Preface

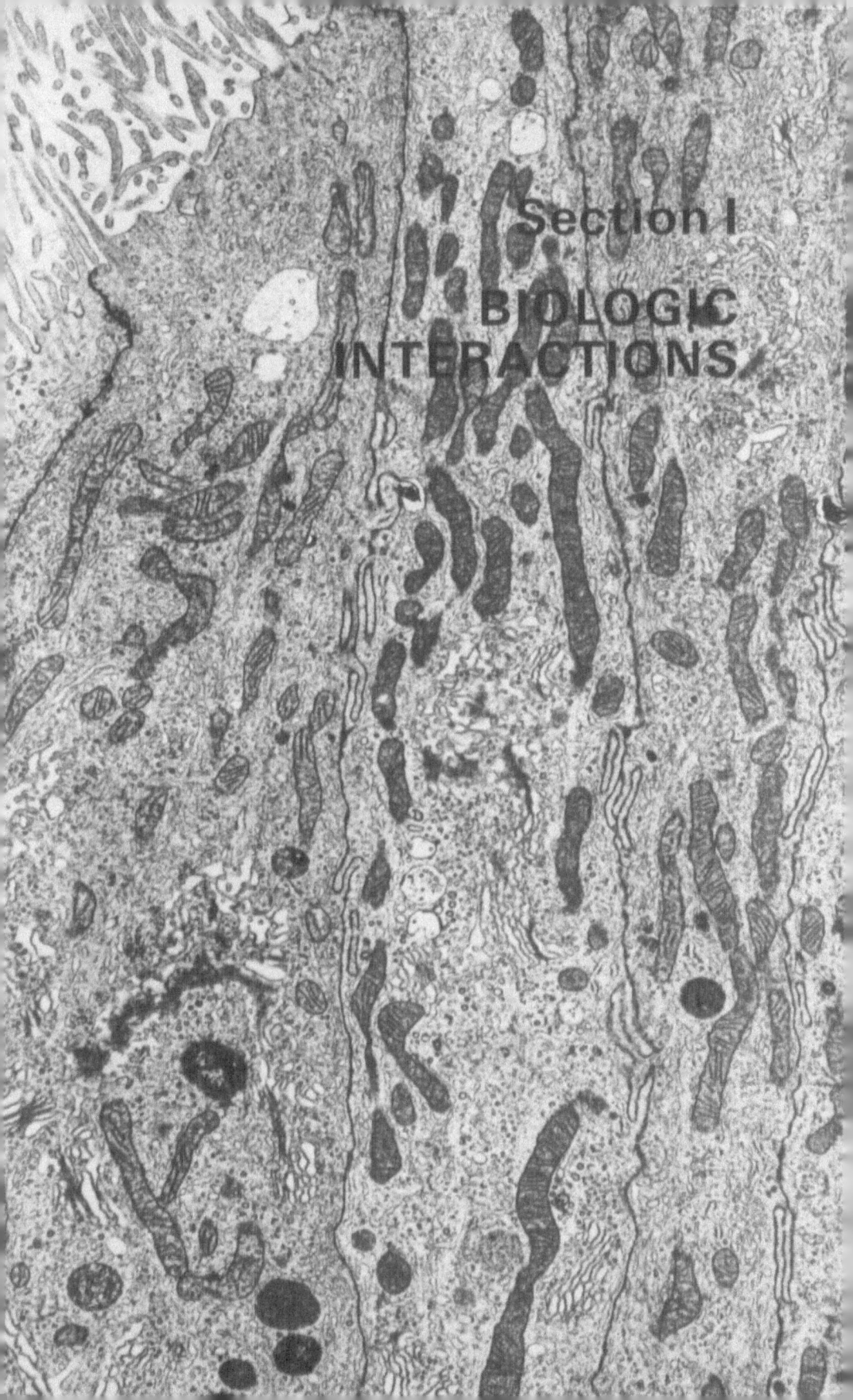

Section I
BIOLOGIC INTERACTIONS

1
Ultrastructure of the decidual response to a progesterone-releasing IUD

U.M. SPORNITZ, K.S. LUDWIG and M. MALL-HAEFELI

INTRODUCTION

The ever-increasing world-wide use of the IUD has prompted intensive research into the physiology of its contraceptive action. From these studies it has become clear that the alterations in morphology as well as in the physiological milieu produced by the IUD are manifold and differ greatly with the type of IUD used.

The inert IUDs, either made of polypropylene or polyethylene (Piotrow *et al.*, 1979) exert their contraceptive action through a foreign body reaction (Moyer and Mishell, 1971; Tatum, 1977). The severity of this foreign body reaction and also some of the side-effects are largely dependent on the size and shape of the IUD (Tatum, 1972). The larger the contact area between the IUD body and the endometrium, the stronger the foreign body reaction and also the undesired side-effects like bleeding, cramping, expulsion, etc. (Piotrow *et al.*, 1979).

The copper IUD is known to produce a foreign body reaction even stronger than that of the inert IUD (Hasson, 1978). Its contraceptive efficacy, however, is apparently amplified through the local effects of copper on the internal milieu of the endometrium, the sperm transport and survival (Hafez, 1980), the inhibition of capacitation (Rosado *et al.*, 1974) and the blastocyst endometrial interaction (El-Badrawi and Hafez, 1980).

In an effort to influence the intrauterine environment and produce fertility control by means of local steroid action, the Progestasert 65, a progesterone therapeutic system for contraception, has been developed (Pharriss *et al.*, 1974). It is a T-shaped device, made of ethylene/vinyl acetate copolymer, which contains a reservoir in the vertical stem with 38 mg of progesterone in a fluid medium (Martinez-Manautou, 1975). The effect of the progesterone released from this IUD on the endometrium is of a rather heterogeneous nature, as has been reported earlier (Spornitz *et al.*, 1980), and depends largely on the localization of the biopsy material with respect to the position of the IUD.

The locally applied progesterone causes severe changes in the morphology

3

and function of the surface epithelium, which are even more pronounced in the glandular epithelium and generally result in irregular or arrested shedding (Ludwig and Spornitz, 1977). These changes (Martinez-Manautou *et al.*, 1975), which include glandular atrophy, suppression of the nucleolar channel system (NCS), impairment of mitochondrial function and the loss of ciliary cells in the surface epithelium, to name only a few, have been reported in detail previously (Spornitz *et al.*, 1980).

Equally important as the changes in the endometrial epithelium are the changes caused through the progesterone IUD in the endometrial stroma (Spornitz *et al.*, 1982).

STROMAL MORPHOLOGY UNDER PHYSIOLOGICAL CONDITIONS

At the beginning of the menstrual cycle the majority of endometrial stroma cells consists of spindle-shaped, poorly differentiated cells, which, like mesenchymal cells, are joined together through slender processes. This stromal cell is one of the target cells of ovarian hormones. It is a rather inconspicuous cell with a narrow rim of cytoplasm, containing not more than a few organelles (Figure 1.1). Under the influence of ovarian hormones these

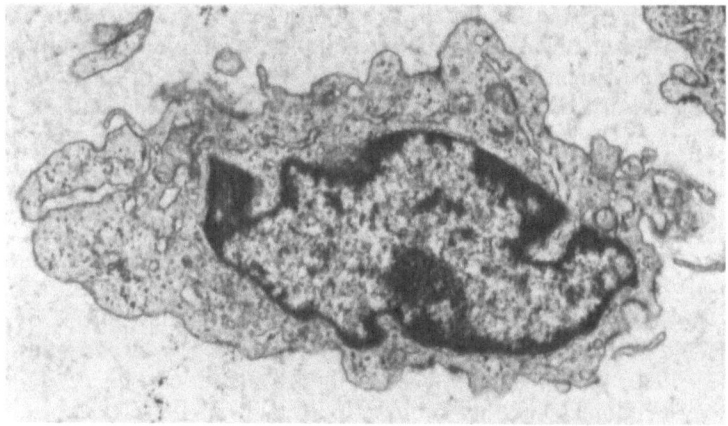

Figure 1.1 Undifferentiated endometrial stroma cell, which is the typical stem cell for the predecidual and decidual cell, during the proliferative phase of the cycle. × 9600

stromal connective tissue cells differentiate into two distinctly different cell types, namely the endometrial granulocytes and the predecidual or pseudodecidual cells (Dallenbach-Hellweg, 1975). At the end of the secretory phase of a cycle about half of the stromal cells have been transformed into predecidual cells (Lawn *et al.*, 1971). These cells possess well-developed organelles and a low ratio of nuclear to cytoplasmic size, i.e. the cells have grown considerably (Figure 1.2). The other half of the stromal cellular elements has been transformed into endometrial granulocytes or K-cells,

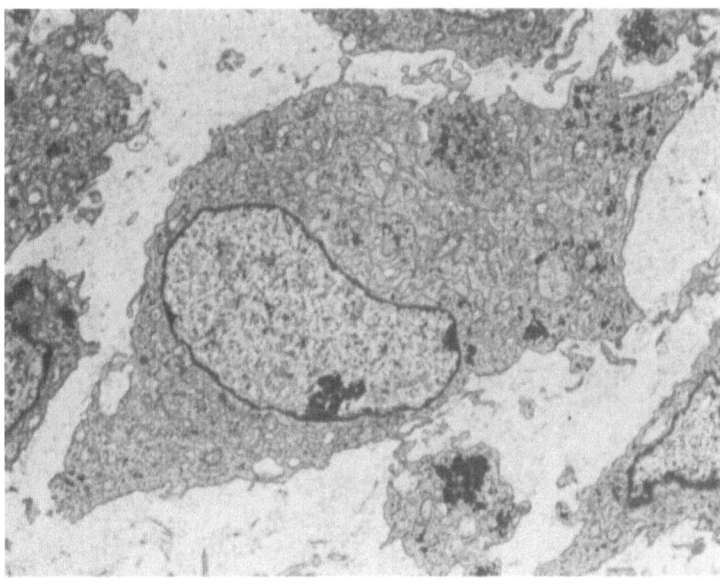

Figure 1.2 Predecidual cell from a biopsy taken at the end of the secretory phase of the pretreatment cycle, when stromal cells are enlarged and their synthetic apparatus is activated. ×4500

which should not be mistaken for leukocytes because of their high content of glycogen and the typical K-cell granules (Figure 1.3). The K-cell granules contain apparently proteolytic enzymes and a phloxinophilic substance closely related to relaxin (Dallenbach and Dallenbach-Hellweg, 1964). In the case of an implantation having occurred the predecidual stroma is then turned into true decidual tissue under the influence of gestational hormones (Wynn, 1974).

LIGHT MICROSCOPY OF THE DECIDUAL RESPONSE

The effect of the locally applied progesterone on the endometrium is all but uniform and therefore whenever possible material obtained through hysterectomy is recommended for investigations. Particularly during the initial phase of an investigation it is advisable to screen the entire uterine cavity by means of light microscopy because of the heterogeneity of the response to the IUD in different parts of the uterine cavity. Thus the morphology of biopsy material can be interpreted much more easily and a better localization of the material with respect to the position of the IUD can be achieved.

With light microscopic sections it can be easily demonstrated that there is a vast difference in morphology between tissue areas in direct contact with the progesterone-releasing vertical stem of the IUD and the other tissue areas.

Already, at the end of the first postinsertion month, the upper third of

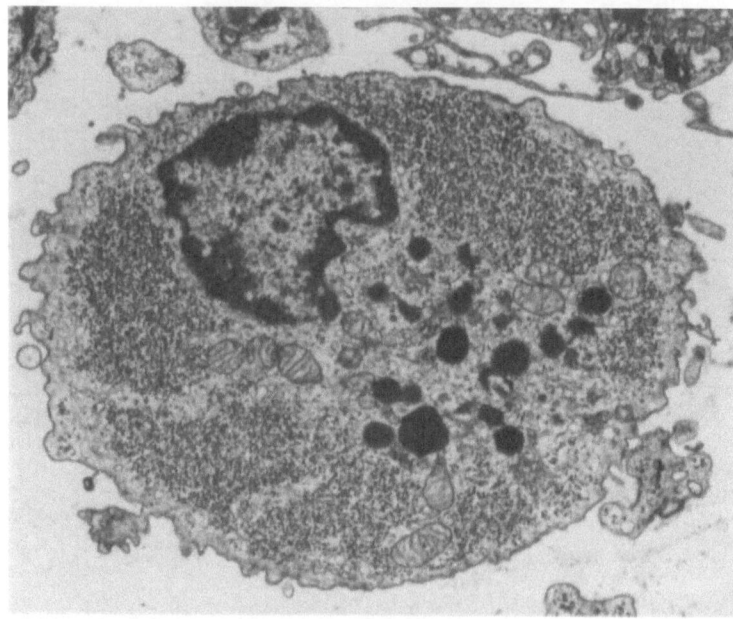

Figure 1.3 Endometrial granulocyte or K-cell which is typical for the late secretory phase of the untreated endometrium. The main features are large amounts of glycogen, an indented nucleus and numerous phloxinophilic granules. The K-cells are never covered by a basal lamina. × 8800

the functionalis, i.e. the zona compacta, which is in direct contact with the IUD, was found to be decidualized. In the more distant parts of the endometrium such a decidualization could not be observed. Periarterial coats were never found, as they are typical for the physiological transformation of the endometrium into decidual tissue. The wave of decidualization apparently started from the stromal areas directly adjoining the vertical stem of the IUD. With longstanding use of the IUD the wave of decidualization spreads into more distant parts of the uterine cavity and is occasionally present even in the region of the tubal openings.

Interestingly enough, however, the decidualization seems to be restricted to the upper part of the functionalis and is hardly ever present in the zona basalis. The areas of the endometrium that were not or not yet transformed into decidual tissue were always found to be moderately edematous regardless of the actual phase of the menstrual cycle.

As an initial response to the progesterone-releasing IUD, during the first few postinsertion months, the decidual cells always show a strongly positive reaction when stained for glycogen. With longstanding use of the IUD the glycogen in the decidual cells is diminished drastically. Similarly, the initial heavy accumulations of Gömöri stain, indicating a large amount of reticular fibres in the intercellular space, are reduced with longstanding use of the Progestasert system.

ELECTRON MICROSCOPY OF THE DECIDUAL RESPONSE

Regardless of the actual phase of the menstrual cycle at which the progesterone-releasing IUD has been inserted, the majority of the cells directly
adjoining the vertical stem of the IUD are invariably already decidualized
at the end of the first postinsertion month. In order to detect cells actually
engaged in the process of decidualization, cells close to but not directly
adjoining the IUD had to be investigated during the first few postinsertion
months. The first notable changes occurring under the influence of the
progesterone-releasing IUD are very similar to those occurring during the
luteal phase of the cycle, resulting in predecidual cells (Figure 1.2). The
nuclear membrane straightens and the nucleus elongates, which is followed
by a growth of the cell. Concomitantly, the synthetic apparatus of the cells
proliferates, particularly the Golgi apparatus and the rough endoplasmic
reticulum. Furthermore, free ribosomes are found all over the cells and the
number of mitochondria is increased. These mitochondria have normally
developed cristae, they are relatively short and measure about 0.3–0.4 μm
in diameter. The endpoint of the development from the inconspicuous
stromal connective tissue cell to the pseudodecidual cell is marked by the
appearance of α- and β-particles of glycogen in the cytoplasm of these cells.
At this point of development the cells are indistinguishable from the predecidual cells occurring at the end of the luteal phase under physiological
conditions. They do possess, however, slender processes which form special-
ized junctions with other pseudodecidualized cells. Under the influence of
the continuous release of progesterone from the IUD these predecidual cells
are then transformed into genuine decidual cells. Although this transformation is rather a continuous process, certain steps involved in this transformation are more obvious than others.

At first large amounts of glycogen appear which, unlike in the pseudodecidual cells, are not loosely distributed over the whole cytoplasm but are
located in rather restricted areas where masses of α-particles or rosettes
form large aggregates, which are so tightly packed that organelles or other
paraplasmatic inclusions are excluded from these areas (Figure 1.4). Subsequent to the formation of the glycogen a massive proliferation of the
Golgi apparatus occurs. On the average longitudinal section through a fully
decidualized cell approximately 10–15 individual dictyosomes can be
counted (Figure 1.4). These dictyosomes are usually located in a juxta-
nuclear position and are hardly ever present in the peripheral cytoplasm.
With progressive decidualization the Golgi apparatus becomes more and
more active, indicated by the appearance of numerous vesicles in the Golgi
area. Some of these vesicles coalesce, thus forming typical multivesicular
bodies (mvbs) (Figure 1.5). Occurring almost simultaneously with the increase in the number of dictyosomes, the rough endoplasmic reticulum also
proliferates and is at first present in the form of somewhat dilated cisternae.
Unlike the Golgi apparatus the rough endoplasmic reticulum cisternae are
distributed over the whole cell and are present even in the peripheral cytoplasm. With longer standing use of the IUD much of the at first cisternal
rough endoplasmic reticulum degranulates, i.e. looses its ribosomes, which

7

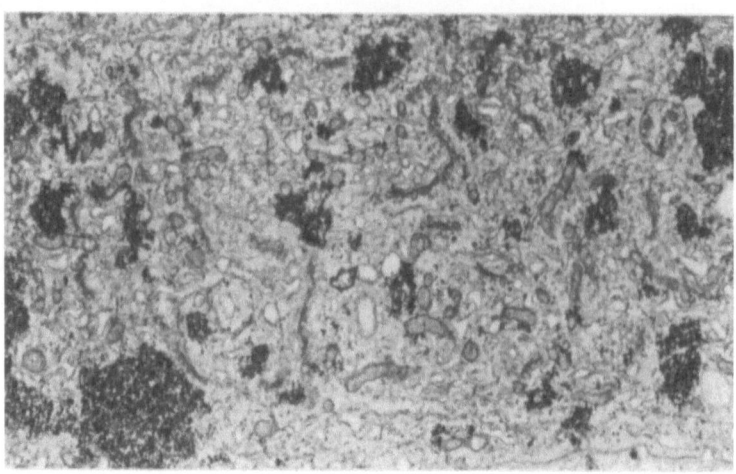

Figure 1.4 Golgi apparatus from a fully activated predecidual cell. The glycogen is distributed over the whole cell in more or less compact aggregates consisting of α-particles. × 11 000

subsequently are found in the form of polysomes or free ribosomes in the cytoplasm. The endoplasmic reticulum then vesiculates so that in the full decidualized cells part of the endoplasmic reticulum is always present in the form of vesicles.

One of the less obvious changes that occur during decidualization involves the mitochondria. Concomitantly occurring with the enormous increase in size of the decidual cells, the total number of mitochondria per individual cell is also increased. This is achieved apparently through budding of new mitochondria, since mitochondria with constrictions and terminal buds can frequently be observed during the phase of decidualization. Subsequent to the budding of new mitochondria, the mitochondria in the decidualizing cells do not grow to regain their original size; they simply elongate, thus reducing greatly their diameter. After several such divisions

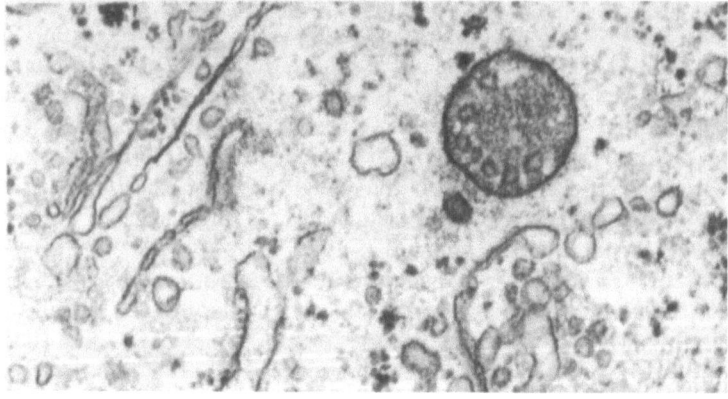

Figure 1.5 Multivesicular body in the Golgi area from a decidualizing cell. Second postinsertion month. × 16 000

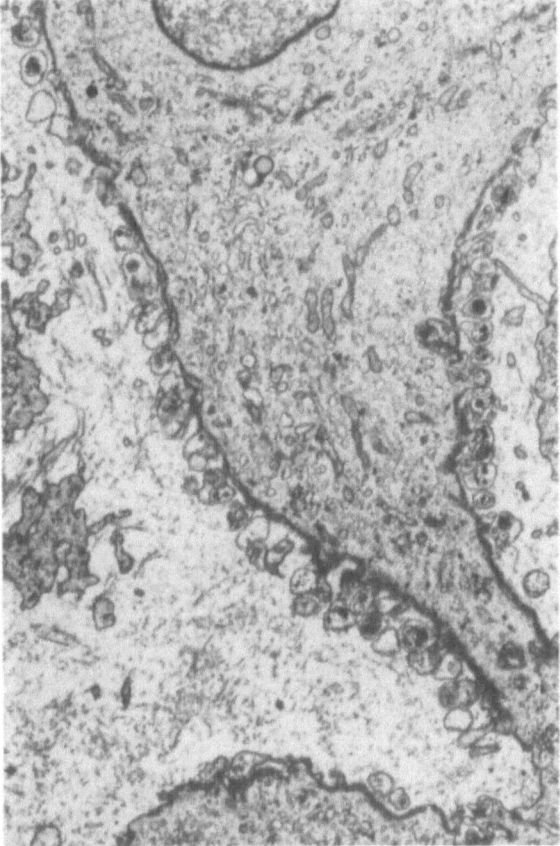

Figure 1.6 Section through a fully decidualized cell on which three of the four characteristic features of decidualized cells can readily be detected: decidual granules, a basal lamina surrounding the cell and miniaturized mitochondria. × 6000

and budding off, of new mitochondria, a minute form of mitochondria results, which is very characteristic for the fully decidualized cell (Figure 1.6). These miniature mitochondria are in fact so typical that they can almost be taken as an indicator for the stage of decidualization, that is the more of the miniature mitochondria measuring approximately 0.15 μm in diameter are present, the more decidualized the cells actually are.

One of the steps indicating the beginning of decidualization of the stromal cells is the dissemination of the aggregated glycogen. Concomitantly occurring with the distribution of the glycogen all over the cytoplasm a partial degradation of the glycogen can be observed. The α-particles are dissolved and much of the glycogen thereafter is present in the form of β-particles. One of the most important events occurring during the course of decidualization is the activation of the Golgi apparatus. With this activation numerous Golgi vesicles are formed as described above which subsequently coalesce to form multivesicular bodies. The mvbs then apparently move to

9

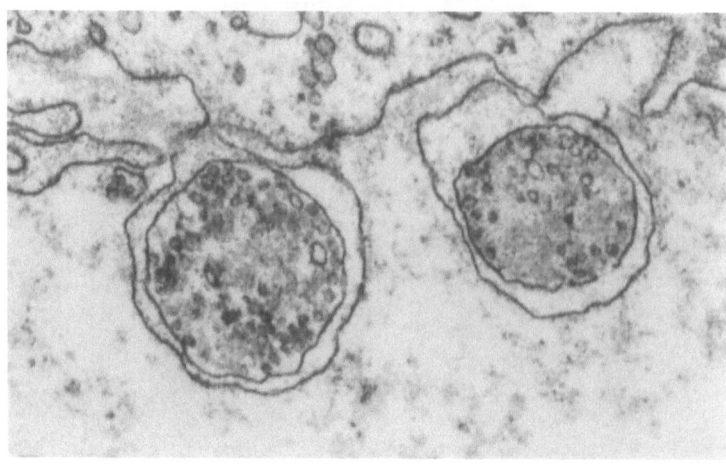

Figure 1.7 Decidual granules in cellular processes protruding from a decidualized cell. Note the rim of cytoplasm surrounding the decidual granules. × 13 000

the periphery to the cells, since shortly after the onset of mvb formation they can be found right underneath the cell membrane. From this hypolemmal position the mvbs move into peduncular processes (Figure 1.7) formed at the surface of the cells which protrude into the intercellular space (Figure 1.8). By the time this occurs some of the multivesicular bodies seem to have attained a somewhat different composition since they are filled with an almost homogeneous osmiophilic content.

Most of the multivesicular bodies, however, do maintain their vesicular nature. The protrusions remain connected to the cell body through a narrow stalk of cytoplasm (Figure 1.9). The cytoplasmic protrusions containing

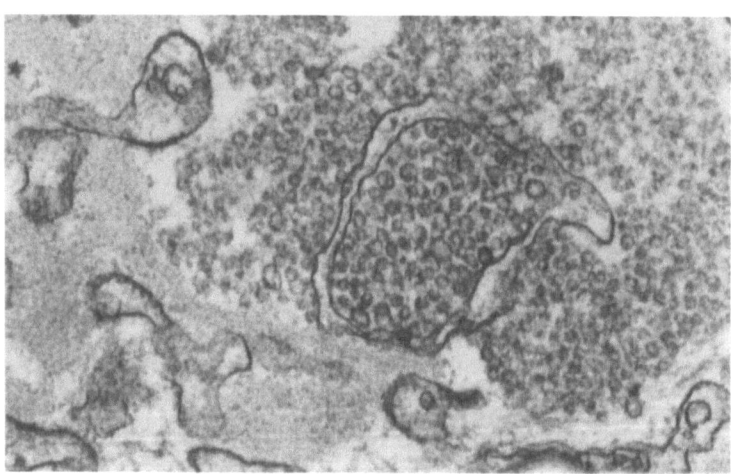

Figure 1.8 Disintegrating decidual granule, discharging its contents into the intercellular space. × 48 000

10

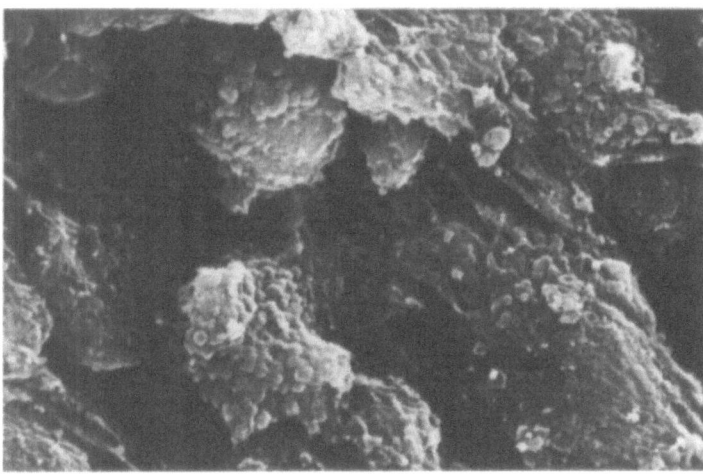

Figure 1.9 Detail of fully decidualized cells showing the typical decidual granules present in the form of beads on the surface of the cells. SEM × 3900

the multivesicular bodies are a unique feature of fully decidualized cells (Figure 1.7). It is suggested, therefore, that they should be called decidual granules. To test the nature of the decidual granules, several cytochemical reactions were carried out. Enzymatic digestion, as performed on ultra-thin sections with proteolytic enzymes (pronase), removed part of the content of the decidual granules. Specific staining for carbohydrates or particularly glycogen yielded negative results. Osmication, on the other hand, indicates a rather high content of unsaturated fatty acids in some of the decidual granules. Fully decidualized cells are covered almost entirely on their surface with the decidual granules which become particularly evident on scanning electron microscopic preparations (Figures 1.9, 1.10). As soon as the decidual cells have started to become synthetically active, indicated by the presence of the large Golgi apparatus and the rough endoplasmic reticulum, an exterior coat very similar to the basement membrane of the glandular cells is formed on the decidual cells (Figure 1.11). Occasionally this basal lamina-like coat, which on the average is about 1500–2000 Å wide, forms a very thick and dense layer which then is up to 6000 Å thick. The basal lamina-like coat covers the decidual cells entirely, except for the places where the decidual granules push through, so that the decidual granules themselves are not covered by a basal lamina. In places where decidual cells are found in direct contact with the surface epithelium or the glandular epithelium, generally the basal lamina underlying the epithelium is continuous with the basal lamina of the decidual cells, which indicates that both are essentially of the same composition. The fully decidualized cell has four very characteristic and unique features which are:

(1)   a large cell body with a highly activated synthetic apparatus,
(2)   miniaturized mitochondria,
(3)   a basal lamina covering the entire surface of the cells,

11

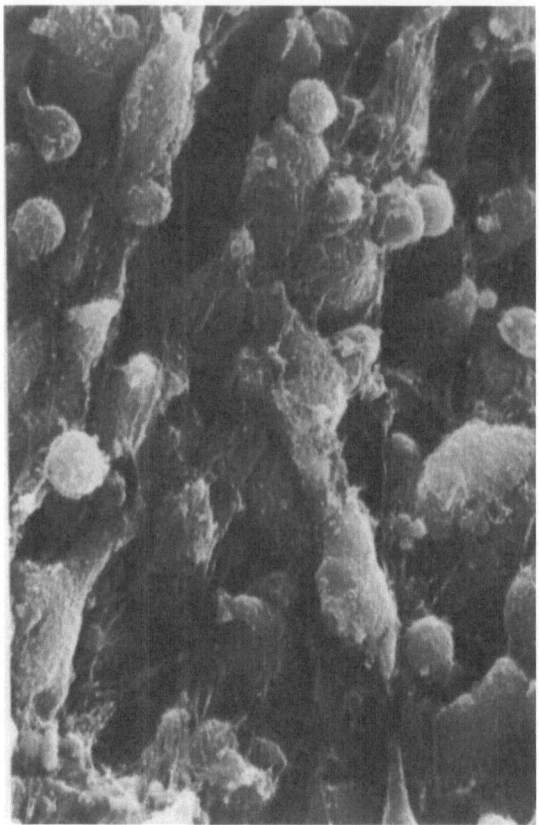

Figure 1.10 Scanning electron microscopic preparation of a decidualized stromal area. The large cells are decidualized cells, the smaller ones are degranulated endometrial granulocytes (K-cells). Note the paucity of connective tissue fibres. SEM × 1400

(4)   and the typical decidual granules protruding from the cell in cyto-
       plasmic processes.

K-CELLS

The K-cells, or endometrial granulocytes (Figure 1.3), which should not be mistaken for leukocytes, as frequently happens, seem to play a role in the process of differentiation of the decidual tissue. They are frequently found in early stages of decidua formation, that is during the first few postinsertion months, to be in intimate contact with the differentiating predecidual cells. At the time when this differentiation starts the K-cells form protrusions which penetrate into deep invaginations on the side of neighbouring predecidual cells. In the normal cycling endometrium such a relationship between K-cells and predecidual cells has never been observed. And in true

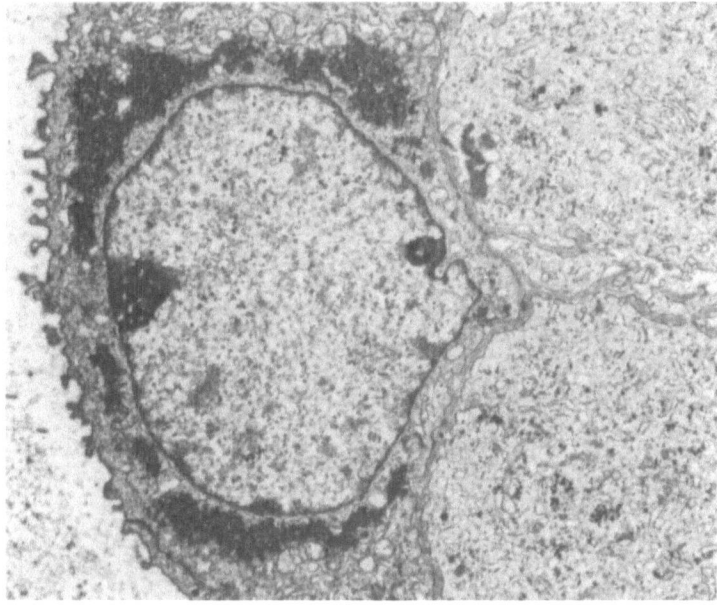

Figure 1.11 Detail from two decidual cells underlying a surface epithelium cell. Note the basal lamina on which the epithelial cell rests, which is continuous with the basal lamina surrounding the two decidual cells. The difference in size between the mitochondria from the epithelial and the mitochondria from the decidual cells is obvious. × 6000

decidual tissue such an observation is difficult to make because electron microscopic investigations during the very first weeks of gestation, when this contact probably occurs, are difficult to carry out for obvious reasons. The penetrating cellular processes form what look like gap junctions with the predecidual cells.

What the exact relationship is between the K-cells and the predecidual cells remains to be elucidated. As a matter of fact, however, both cells go through various stages of differentiation after this contact has occurred. This leads, on the side of the predecidual cells, to the formation of decidual cells. The K-cells, on the other side, subsequently degranulate and discharge large amounts of glycogen into the intercellular space by detaching parts of their cytoplasm in a way very similar to the mode of formation of blood platelets (Figure 1.12). From both, the degranulation and the detaching of cytoplasmic areas, a cell type results, which very closely resembles the stem cell found under physiological conditions during the early proliferative phase of the cycle, from which the K-cells originate.

Since most other cells are decidual cells, both cell types can very easily be distinguished from one another. This is also very easily done on scanning electron microscopic preparations because of the vast difference in size (Figure 1.10). In fully decidualized tissue areas the number of K-cells containing relaxin granules is thus drastically reduced.

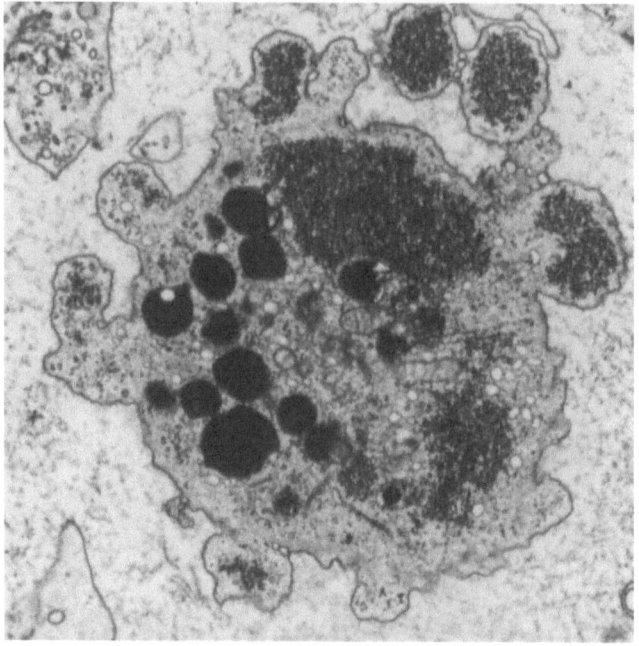

Figure 1.12 Disintegrating K-cell which is discharging glycogen by detaching peripheral areas of cytoplasm. ×9800

LONGSTANDING USE OF THE PROGESTERONE-RELEASING IUD

Already during the process of decidualization decidual granules can be observed which have been secreted into the intercellular space where they disintegrate thus contributing to the mass of intercellular substance which is formed during the decidualization of the endometrial stroma (Figure 1.8). With longstanding use of the IUD the majority of the decidual granules is released into the intercellular space, so that decidual cells are frequently completely degranulated. This degranulation leaves behind only the stalks by means of which the granules were connected to the decidual cells. The decidual granules themselves are usually not of a uniform size but vary between 0.4 and 0.9 μm in diameter (Figures 1.6, 1.8). In most of the observed cases the decidual granules are secreted into the intercellular space together with the process of cytoplasm in which they are contained. Since this cytoplasmic bud also varies in size, usually different amounts of cytoplasm are pinched off together with the decidual granules. Thus the content of the decidual granules is surrounded by two membranes, that is the cytoplasmic membrane and the membrane of the multivesicular body or osmiophilic body itself. With longer standing use of the IUD many of these secreted granules disintegrate, including not only the dissolution of the outer membrane, but also the dissolution of the multivesicular body

14

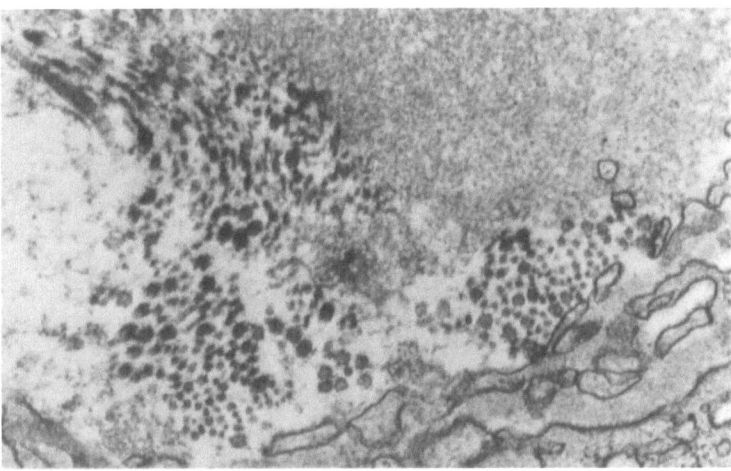

Figure 1.13 Collagen fibers and fibrinoid. There is a sharp borderline between the areas occupied by either material. × 32 000

membrane itself. Frequently decidual granules are present which do not only have a discontinuous membrane but which are also surrounded by numerous vesicles and osmiophilic substance which apparently has been released from the decidual granules. The further away this material is located from the decidual granule, the more the individual vesicle seems to be dissolving, thus contributing to the mass of intercellular substance which in most areas has a morphology very similar to the fibrinoid of the utero-placental interface (Figure 1.13).

In the areas where there appears to be a massive secretion of decidual granules into the intercellular space the amount of collagen is drastically diminished as compared to predecidual tissue. There is, in fact, a reciprocal relationship between the amount of collagen and fibrinoid present in the decidual areas, in such a way that, with the progression of the decidualization, the fibrinoid predominates. Fibrinoid and collagen do not mix very well with one another; they are almost mutually exclusive. The borderline between the areas with collagen and the areas with fibrinoid is very pronounced (Figure 1.13). Fibrin in turn can frequently be found to have formed aggregates with the fibrinoid, particularly in areas where, due to vascular damage, red blood cells have entered the stroma. In uteri where the decidualization is particularly pronounced a unique structure, namely collagen vacuoles, can be observed (Figure 1.14). The first collagen vacuoles are probably simple cytoplasmic invaginations containing some of the adhering collagen fibers. In later stages, however, the collagen vacuoles are fully internalized parts of the extracellular space (Figure 1.15), as could be demonstrated by means of serial sections. Even in cases where the collagen vacuoles were found in the peripheral cytoplasm, close to the plasmalemm, they were clearly distinguishable from invaginations since they were never lined by a coat of basal lamina-like material (Figure 1.14), like other simple

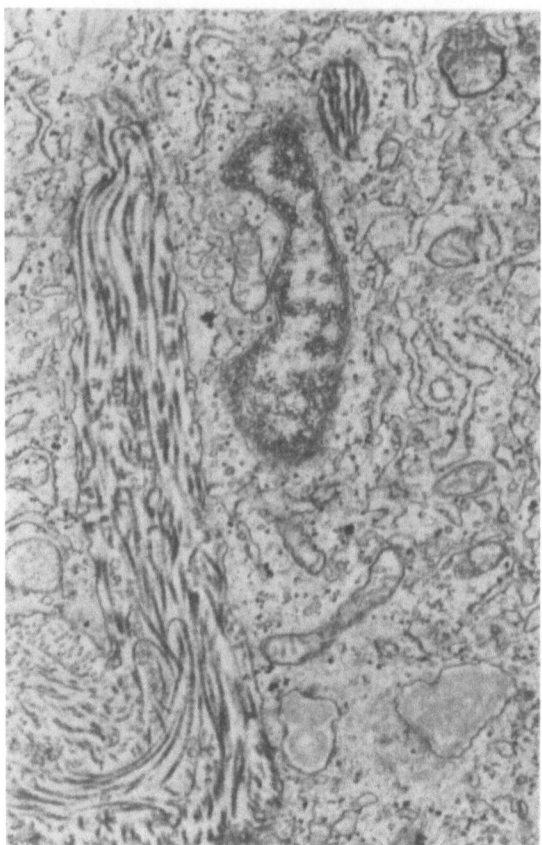

Figure 1.14 Collagen vacuole in an arrested decidual cell. The vacuole itself is not lined by a basal lamina like the two invaginations in the lower right part of the micrograph. There are several vesicular structures inside the vacuole. × 26 000

invaginations. With longstanding use of the progesterone-releasing IUD the collagen vacuoles increase in size, lysosomes are incorporated into the vacuoles and the collagen fibers themselves become less clearly visible as they are being digested. Occasionally, decidual cells can be encountered which are suggestive of unloading the more or less digested content of the collagen vacuoles into the intercellular space. Scanning electron micrographs disclose that fully decidualized cells remain in contact with one another through cytoplasmic extension (Figure 1.10). These extensions are incorporated into invaginations. With longstanding use of the progesterone-releasing IUD the collagen vacuoles increase in size, lysosomes are incorporated into the vacuoles and the collagen fibers themselves become less clearly visible as they are being digested. Occasionally, decidual cells can be encountered which

Because of the extensive decidualization of the upper layer of the functionalis much of the decidualized tissue is not shed during the menstrual cycle but remains within the uterine cavity. This tissue which does not

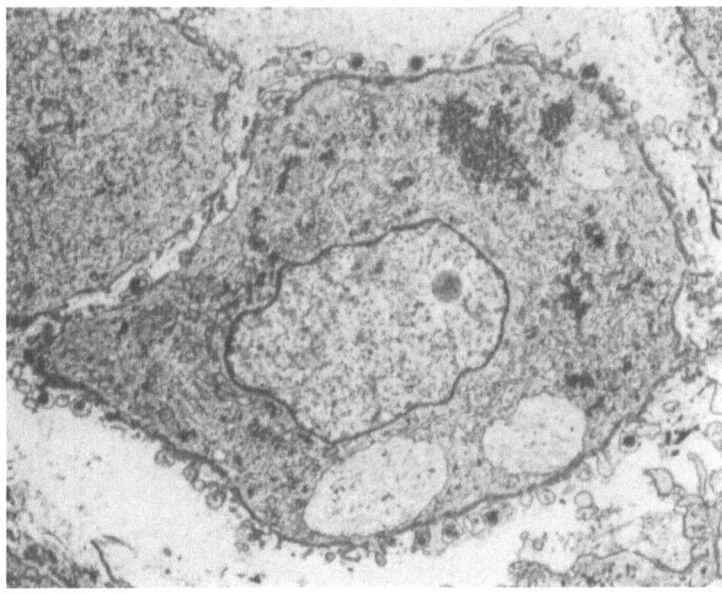

Figure 1.15 Late or arrested decidual cell with a few remaining decidual granules, basal lamina and three collagen vacuoles which appear almost empty, since there are only a very few solid fibers present. × 4800

participate in the desquamation develops a rather rigid appearance with longstanding use of the IUD. The cells resemble decidualized cells in many respects, but they do not possess any decidual granules. They are surrounded by large amounts of fibrinoid which is merging with their basal lamina. These cells have depleted their glycogen stores and reduced their synthetic activity drastically. The mitochondria remain unchanged, i.e. they are still very numerous and much smaller than usual mitochondria.

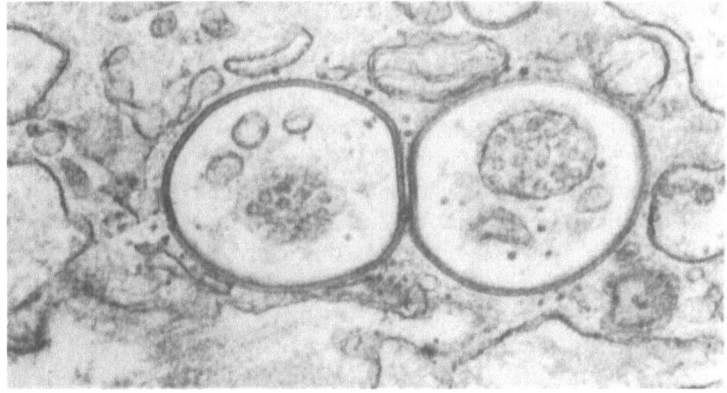

Figure 1.16 Anular cell junctions (gap junction?) between two decidual cells. The membranes in these junctions appear to be pentalaminar. × 60 000

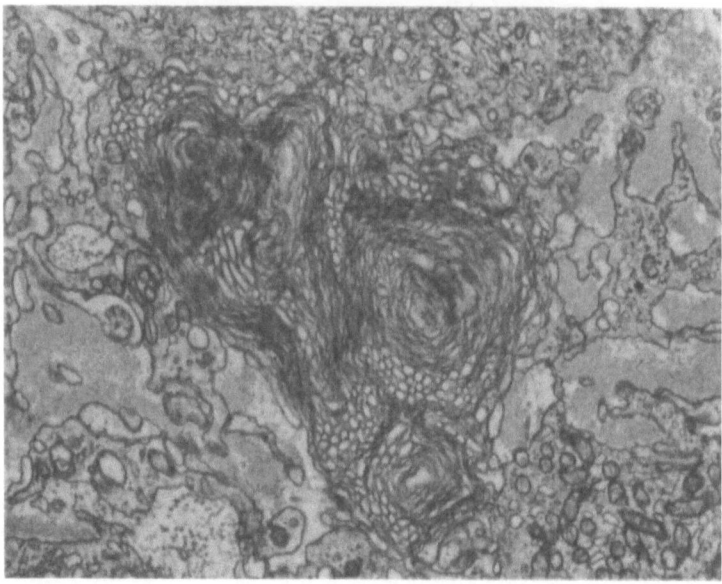

Figure 1.17 Aggregates of endoplasmic reticulum in a hyperstimulated decidual cell during the 12th postinsertion month. These aggregates are part of a stromal Arias-Stella reaction. Note the large amount of fibrinoid present in the intercellular space. × 6000

ARIAS-STELLA REACTION

On light microscopical level, the first signs of an Arias-Stella reaction generally appear in the glandular epithelium, where they become easily visible because of an enormous growth of the nuclei and a voluminous clear cytoplasm. With the progesterone-releasing IUD the first signs of an Arias-Stella reaction can be observed in the decidualized stromal cells. The reaction apparently starts in the cells lying directly underneath the vertical stem of the IUD particularly those which are in direct contact with the surface epithelium. The areas of the surface epithelium appear to be thinning out and the decidual cells correspond in the their morphology with the type of decidual cells occurring after longstanding use of the IUD, i.e. they do not possess any decidual granules and their synthetic apparatus, namely the Golgi apparatus and the endoplasmic reticulum, appears to be rather inactive. With the onset of the Arias-Stella reaction the miniaturized mitochondria of these cells proliferate, so that cells can be found which are almost completely filled with mitochondria. The most obvious sign of the stromal Arias-Stella reaction, however, is the formation of large whorls of smooth endoplasmic reticulum (Figure 1.17), which sometimes occupy as much as 25% of the cell. These endoplasmic reticulum whorls frequently have a myelin-like configuration. With progressive decidualization the myelin-like accumulations show signs of degeneration like coalescence of individual membranes and the formation of osmiophilic whorls.

The remaining endoplasmic reticulum which is not incorporated into the whorls also degranulates, i.e. it loses its ribosomes and becomes dilated so that much of the cytoplasm of these cells is occupied by endoplasmic reticulum either in the form of whorls or in the form of small vesicles.

DISCUSSION

The decidualization of the endometrial stroma is a local effect produced by the progesterone released from the IUD. This is clearly demonstrated through the fact that the decidualization starts and progresses from the areas in direct contact with the IUD and that there are no periarterial coats of decidualized cells. This does not, of course, imply that there is no systemic effect at all, particularly since evidence collected in recent years strongly supports the theory of such systemic effects, like changes in the oviduct (Spornitz et al., 1980), the rise of serum prolactin levels in lactating woman (Badraoui et al., 1981) and the altered corpus luteum function in lactating woman (Abdalla et al., 1981).

Through the addition of progesterone to the inert IUD, the contraceptive efficacy has been greatly improved (Pharriss et al., 1974). Much of the improved safety is a result of the progesterone acting on the glandular epithelium causing either glandular atrophy (Spornitz et al., 1980; Wan et al., 1977) or arrested and irregular secretion (Ludwig and Spornitz, 1977; Hagenfeldt et al., 1977). Through the asynchronous development of the uterine glands the endometrium is not prepared for the implantation of the blastocyst. The human endometrium is apparently best prepared for the implantation of the blastocyst between the 18th and 21st day of the cycle (Scommegna et al., 1974) when the predecidual reaction is still completely absent (Noyes et al., 1950). Very little is known about the possible effects of a stromal predecidual reaction on the implantation itself. For the initial steps of implantation the predecidual reaction is certainly not a prerequisite. The fact, that the predecidual reaction normally appears only after the optimum period for an implantation has passed, does not necessarily imply that the predecidual reaction itself is detrimental to implantation. As far as the genuine decidual reaction is concerned, however, there appears to be little, if any, doubt that it can act effectively as a barrier against the implantation of a blastocyst. Therefore, not only the altered morphology of the glandular epithelium, i.e. its asynchronous development, but also the decidual reaction of the stroma should be considered part of the contraceptive action of the progesterone IUD.

Although the transformation from the predecidual to the decidual cells is a gradual one, involving several intermediate steps, both the predecidual and the decidual cell are distinctly different entities and should not be mistaken for one another as often happens. It should be clearly pointed out again, that only the cells with decidual granules, a basal lamina and miniaturized mitochondria can be considered true decidual cells. For the identification of all three parameters it is necessary to use the electron microscope.

The ultrastructure of the cells decidualized under the influence of the progesterone from the IUD is in most details identical with the ultrastructure of true decidual cells (Lawn *et al.*, 1971; Liebig and Stegner, 1977; Wynn, 1974; Spornitz, unpublished observations).

The decidual granules are a characteristic feature of genuine decidual cells. They are even found in the ectopic decidual cells of the ovarian cortex at term (Herr *et al.*, 1978, 1979). Decidual granules can be divided into two groups on the basis of their morphology, one group with a clearly vesicular content and the other group with a strongly osmiophilic nature. The latter type of decidual granules resembles very much secretory products formed in granulosa lutein cells (Booher *et al.*, 1981). In the granulosa lutein cells these secretory granules are believed to be related to hormone secretion.

On the basis of morphology alone it is difficult if not impossible to compare the intercellular substance present in the decidualized stroma with the fibrinoid of the uteroplacental interface. However, the similarity with fibrinoid from mature placentas (Azab *et al.*, 1972; Sutcliffe *et al.*, 1982) is striking and it would seem logical that the progesterone induced decidual cells secrete similar products as do the decidual cells induced through implantation.

Collagen vacuoles, as they occur with longstanding use of the IUD, resemble very much those described in regressing decidual cells towards the end of pregnancy (Dallenbach-Hellweg, 1961), in the non-pregnant uterus (Dyer and Peppler, 1976) and in the rat uterus up to 6 days postpartum (Schwarz and Güldner, 1967). There is, however, a major difference, namely that the collagen vacuoles described in this chapter occur in stromal cells actively engaged in the process of decidualization. They are a sign of collagen breakdown rather than synthesis, since with progressing decidualization they become more and more filled with lysosome-like particles. It is only in the more or less static decidual cells, occurring with longstanding use of the IUD, that they seem to be discharging their contents into the intercellular space, thus also participating in the formation of intercellular substance.

The endometrial granulocytes or K-cells are known to be dependent upon an absolute or relative deficiency of progesterone which stimulates the discharge of their relaxin-containing granules (Dallenbach-Hellweg, 1975). The exact nature of the stimulus for the disintegration of these cells in the immediate surrounding of the IUD remains to be elucidated, since it certainly cannot be a lack of progesterone. The discharge of the relaxin granules is believed to lead to a dissolution of reticular fibers, which in turn alleviates the implantation of the blastocyst (Dallenbach-Hellweg *et al.*, 1965). This is corroborated by our own findings, namely that the amount of material stainable with the Gömöri stain is drastically reduced concomitantly with the degranulation of the endometrial granulocytes.

The Arias-Stella reaction is of particular interest. It is known to be dependent on the presence of chorionic tissue (Arias-Stella, 1954), but can also be provoked by clomiphene therapy (Bernhardt *et al.*, 1966). In most cases the morphology of the glandular epithelium is the sole basis for the diagnosis of an Arias-Stella reaction (ASR), which is considered to be sufficient even when a decidual reaction is missing (Mackles *et al.*, 1961;

Frederiksen, 1958). The attempts to use the ASR as an indicator for ectopic pregnancy have failed to succeed, particularly because of the absence of a pronounced ASR in many biopsies (Pildes and Wheeler, 1957; Mackles *et al.*, 1961). Because of the limitations of the light microscope to detect subcellular changes, stromal cells have in most cases been disregarded with respect to ASR. As has been demonstrated in the factual part of this chapter there is a drastic stromal ASR caused through the locally applied progesterone. In contrast to the stromal reaction, the epithelial reaction is not very pronounced. Moreover, the stromal reaction is present in most cases in patients who have a highly decidualized endometrium and who have also used the IUD for periods close to or even longer than 12 months. Thus the ASR can, in the case of the progesterone-releasing IUD, probably be regarded as resulting from a high endogenous level of hormones combined with high rates of progesterone released from the IUD. Because of the importance of the ASR with respect to a possible ectopic pregnancy, this phenomenon should not be neglected even in the case of ASR occurring in patients with a progesterone IUD. There might even be a connection between the uterine ASR and ectopic pregnancy in such a way that the presence of ASR alleviates ectopic implantation, as the rate of ectopic pregnancy comes up to about 50% of the total number of pregnancies under the progesterone IUD (Zador *et al.*, 1976). In conclusion, we would like to emphasize that the decidualization of the endometrium under the progesterone-releasing IUD, although far from being uniform, is identical to the formation of true decidua during gestation. This fact deserves our attention not only because the decidualization is part of the contraceptive effect but also because with the progesterone IUD we have an ideal model at hand to study the maternal contribution to the formation of the decidua.

ACKNOWLEDGEMENTS

The authors wish to thank Mr. R. Betschart and Mr. G. Morson for their excellent technical assistance and Mr H. Stöcklin for the photographic work.

Part of this study has been supported by a grant from Ciba–Geigy Stiftung to UMS, which is gratefully acknowledged.

References

Abdalla, M.I., Ibrahim, I.I., Osman, M.I., Badraoui, M.H.H. and Askalani, H. (1981). Corpus luteum function in lactating women using the progestasert-system. *Contracept. Deliv. Syst.*, **2**, 127-32

Arias-Stella, J. (1954). Atypical endometrial changes associated with the presence of chorionic tissue. *Am. Med. Assoc. Arch. Pathol.*, **58**, 112-28

Azab, I., Okamura, H. and Beer, A. (1972). Decidual cell production of human placental fibrinoid. *Obstet. Gynecol.*, **40**, 186-93

Badraoui, M.H.H., Askalani, H., Mahrous, I., Osman, M.I., Bayad, M.A.B., Ibrahim, I.I. and Abdalla, M.I. (1981). Serum prolactin levels in lactating women using the progestasert-system. *Contracept. Deliv. Syst.*, **2**, 121-6

Bernhardt, R.N., Bruns, P.D. and Drose, V. (1966). Atypical endometrium associated with ectopic pregnancy. *Obstet. Gynecol.*, **28**, 849-53

Booher, C., Enders, A.C., Hendricks, A.G. and Hess, D.L. (1981). Structural characteristics of the corpus luteum during implantation of the Rhesus monkey (Macaca mulatta). *Am. J. Anat.*, **160**, 17-36

Dallenbach, F.D. and Dallenbach-Hellweg. G. (1964). Immunohistologische Untersuchungen zur Lokalisation des Relaxins in menschlicher Placenta und Decidua. *Virchows Arch. Pathol. Anat.*, **337**, 301-16

Dallenbach-Hellweg, G. (1961). Ueber die Rückbildung von Deciduazellen unter Auftreten von Kollageneinschlüssen. *Virchows Arch. Pathol. Anat.*, **334**, 195-206

Dallenbach-Hellweg, G. (1975). *Histopathology of the Endometrium.* (Berlin: Springer Verlag)

Dallenbach-Hellweg, G., Battista, J.V. and Dallenbach, F.D. (1965). Immunohistological and histochemical localization of relaxin in the metrial gland of the pregnant rat. *Am. J. Anat.*, **117**, 433-50

Dyer, R.F. and Peppler, R.B. (1976). Intercellular collagen in the nonpregnant and IUD-containing rat uterus. *Anat. Rec.*, **187**, 241-8

El-Badrawi, H.H. and Hafez, E.S.E. (1980). Physiological mechanisms of IUDs. In Hafez, E.S.E. and van Os, W.A.A. (eds.) *Medicated Intrauterine Devices*, pp. 60-83. (The Hague: Martinus Nijhoff)

Frederiksen, T. (1958). The Arias-Stella reaction as an aid in the diagnosis of ectopic pregnancy. *Acta Obstet. Gynecol. Scand.*, **37**, 86-96

Hafez, E.S.E. (1980). Mode of action of inert, copper and steroid-releasing IUDs. *Contracept. Deliv. Syst.*, **1**, 206-9

Hagenfeldt, K., Landgren, B.A., Edström, K. and Johannisson, E. (1977). Biochemical and morphological changes in the human endometrium induced by the Progestasert device. *Contraception*, **16**, 183-97

Hasson, H.M. (1978). Copper IUDs. *J. Reprod. Med.*, **20**, 139-54

Herr, J.C., Heidger, P.M., Scott, J.R., Anderson, J.W., Curet, L.B. and Mossmann, H.W. (1978). Decidual cells in the human ovary at term. I. Incidence, gross anatomy and ultrastructural features of merocrine secretion. *Am. J. Anat.*, **152**, 7-28

Herr, J.C., Platz, C.E., Heidger, P.M. and Curet, L.B. (1979). Smooth muscle within ovarian decidual nodules: a link to leiomyomatosis peritonealis disseminata? *Obstet. Gynecol.*, **53**, 451-5

Lawn, A.M., Wilson, E.W. and Finn, C.A. (1971). The ultrastructure of human decidual and predecidual cells. *J. Reprod. Fertil.*, **26**, 85-90

Liebig, W. and Stegner, H.E. (1977). Decidualisation of the endometrial stromal cell. *Arch. Gynäkol.*, **223**, 19-31

Ludwig, K.S. and Spornitz, U.M. (1977). Veränderungen des Endometriums beim Progestasert-System. *Acta Anat.*, **99**, 237

Mackles, A., Wolfe, S.A. and Pozner, S.N. (1961). Cellular atypia in endometrial glands (Arias-Stella reaction) as an aid in the diagnosis of ectopic pregnancy. *Am J. Obstet. Gynecol.*, **81**, 1209-19

Martinez-Manautou, J. (1975). Contraception by intrauterine release of progesterone. Clinical results. *J. Steroid Biochem.*, **6**, 889-94

Martinez-Manautou, J., Maqueo, M., Aznar, R., Pharriss, B.B. and Zaffaroni, A. (1975). Endometrial morphology in woman exposed to uterine systems releasing progesterone. *Am. J. Obstet. Gynecol.*, **121**, 175

Moyer, D.L. and Mishell, D.R. (1971). Reactions of human endometrium to the intrauterine foreign body. 2. Long-term effects on the endometrial histology and cytology. *Am. J. Obstet. Gynecol.*, **111**, 66-80

Noyes, R.W., Hertig, A.T. and Rock, I. (1950). Dating the endometrial biopsy. *Fertil. Steril.*, **1**, 3-25

Pharriss, B.B., Erickson, R., Baskaw, J., Hoff, S., Place, V.A. and Zaffaroni, A. (1974). Progestasert: a uterine therapeutic system for long-term contraception. 1. Philosophy and clinical efficacy. *Fertil. Steril.*, **25**, 915-21

Pildes, R.B. and Wheeler, J.D. (1957). Atypical cellular changes in endometrial glands associated with ectopic pregnancy. *Am. J. Obstet. Gynecol.*, **73**, 79-88

Piotrow, P.T., Rinehart, W. and Schmidt, J.C. (1979). IUDs—update on safety, effectiveness and research. *Population Reports*, Series B, Number 3

Rosado, A., Hicks, J.J., Aznar, R. and Mercado, E. (1974). Intrauterine contraception with

Progesterone-T device—interference with metabolic-activity and capacitation of spermatozoa. *Contraception*, **9**, 39–51

Schwarz, W. and Güldner, F.H. (1967). Elektronenmikroskopische Untersuchungen des Kollagenabbaus im Uterus der Ratte nach Schwangerschaft. *Z. Zellforsch.*, **83**, 416–26

Scommegna, A.A., Avila, T., Luna, M., Rao, R. and Dmowski, P. (1974). Fertility control by intrauterine release of progesterone. *Obstet. Gynecol.*, **43**, 769–79

Spornitz, U.M., Ludwig, K.S. and Mall-Haefeli, M. (1982). Ultrastructure of decidual response to Progestasert IUD. Presented at the *Reproductive Health Care Symposium*, October 1982, Maui, Hawaii, USA

Spornitz, U.M., Ludwig, K.S., Mall-Haefeli, M., Werner-Zodrow, I. and Uettwiller, A. (1980). The effect of the progesterone releasing IUD on the morphology of the endometrium and the oviduct. In Hafez, E.S.E. and van Os, W.A.A. (eds.) *Medicated Intrauterine Devices*, pp. 44–54. (The Hague: Martinus Nijhoff)

Sutcliffe, R.G., Davies, M., Hunter, J.B., Waters, J.J. and Parry, J.E. (1982). The protein composition of the fibrinoid material at the human uteroplacental interface. *Placenta*, **3**, 297–308

Tatum, H.J. (1972). Intrauterine contraception. *Am. J. Obsetet. Gynecol.*, **112**, 1001–23

Tatum, H.J. (1977). Clinical aspects of intrauterine contraception. Circumspection 1976. *Fertil. Steril.*, **28**, 3–28

Wan, L.S., Hsu, Y.C., Ganguly, M. and Bigelow, B. (1977). Effect of the Progestasert on the menstrual pattern, ovarian steroids and endometrium. *Contraception*, **16**, 417–33

Wynn, R.M. (1974). Ultrastructural development of the human decidua. *Am. J. Obstet. Gynecol.*, **118**, 652–70

Zador, G., Nilsson, B.A., Nilsson, B., Sjöberg, N.O., Westrom, L. and Wiese, J. (1976). Clinical experience with the uterine progesterone system (Progestasert). *Contraception*, **13**, 559–71

2
Effects of copper IUDs on cervical cytology and influences on transtubal sperm migration

U. J. KOCH

GENERAL COMMENTS

In the last two decades, the proportion of intrauterine contraception has constantly increased in importance. As part of the foreign body reaction of the endometrium multiple morphopathological and pathophysiological changes could be observed, which individually and/or in combination are responsible for IUD's mode of action. The primary result of the foreign body reaction is endometrial leukocytosis together with biochemical and enzymic changes of the intrauterine milieu. Alterations in the composition of the fluids of the female genital tract may disturb gamete transport and interrupt embryonic growth during preimplantation and postimplantation periods (Moyer *et al.*, 1979; Moyer and Shaw, 1980). In the presence of an IUD, biochemical, biophysical, cytological and histological changes of the epithelia and their fluids have been observed. In addition, influences on the myometrial contractability are possible, together with influences on tubal peristalsis. All IUDs act as foreign bodies in the intrauterine cavity, causing a sterile inflammatory response of the endometrium as long as the IUD remains in place. This reaction is similar to other foreign body reactions. A typical symptom of this reaction is leukocytosis in the fluids of the uterine cavity and cervix. In relation to the medication of the IUDs, the reaction of the female genital tract including the side-effects are modified. The injury of tissue cells, caused by the IUD, leads to a release of proteases which are able to activate collagenolysis and to produce polypeptides by digestive mechanisms. The collagenolysis and polypeptides initiate the migration of neutrophils from the blood vessels by chemotaxis. The increased density of leukocytes in the endometrium and its fluids modifies significantly the milieu of the uterine cavity. Together with neutrophils, macrophages and foreign body giant cells have been seen. The leukocytes are responsible for the increase of the myometrial activity and oviductal peristalsis, stimulated by prostaglandins (Myatt *et al.*, 1977), which these cells produce. The leukocytes are also important for the increase of fibrinolytic activity by proteolysis and for the hostile environment for gametes and the blastocyst by cytolysis. Inhibition of implantation, embryotoxic effects, disturbances of DNA metabolism, and phagocytosis of the cell components, the ovum, the blastocyst and the spermatozoa, were observed. Inhibition of fertility is the result of the IUD's multifactorial mode of action.

The following questions are to be discussed: Are precancerous changes induced by IUDs? Are there influences of menstrual hygiene and/or sexual activity on cervical cytology? What is the distribution of the cytological results in the different methods of contraception especially in combination with menstrual hygiene? With which method of contraception is the risk of contracting an inflammatory vaginal disease the highest? Do the changes of the intrauterine milieu cause disturbances of the transport of spermatozoa and/or the oocytes, or is the most important factor of IUD's mode of action the inhibition of implantation of the blastocyst?

CERVICAL CYTOLOGY IN USERS OF DIFFERENT METHODS OF FERTILITY REGULATION

The basic problem in the comparative cytological diagnostics of the individual contraceptive groups is the composition of the various cohorts, which often do not allow comparative statistical analysis. In the past, many investigations in this field were performed and cancerous influences due to the use of oral contraceptives and intrauterine devices were discussed. In the majority of the publications cancer-inducing effects of oral contraceptives and intrauterine devices could not be proven. Women using oral contraceptives or intrauterine devices or barrier methods with spermicides belong, in principle, from the sexual behavior pattern and from social surroundings, to different groups. Especially influences of pregnancies dependent upon age should be regularly considered. It must be emphasized, that there are no strict divisions of the different groups, only artificial divisions in the statistics. In addition, it can be normally observed, that most women often change contraceptive methods for various reasons, so that long-term effects on cervical cytology are difficult to assess.

INFLUENCES OF AGE AND MENSTRUAL HYGIENE ON CERVICAL CYTOLOGY

According to the statistical investigations of cancer detection screening, published by Soost and Baur (1980), cervical cancer can be observed starting with the 19th year of age. The rate of invasive cancer of the uterine cervix increases from $0.1-0.2\%_{oo}$ in young women to $0.9\%_{oo}$ in women of 55-59 years of age and reaches a maximum of $2.7\%_{oo}$ in old women. The highest rate of carcinoma *in situ* and severe dysplasia was seen between the ages of 25 and 29 with $2.9\%_{oo}$. The mild and moderate dysplasia reached their maximum of circa $1\%_{oo}$ around the age of 24 and declined continuously to below $0.2\%_{oo}$ with increasing age. The duration of carcinogenesis is assumed to be a period of 15-20 years according to Boyes (1975). The peak of precancerous changes can be observed between the ages of 25 and 29 years according to the results of most of the investigators (Bibbo *et al.*, 1971; Boyes, 1975; Soost and Baur, 1980). Without regard to race-specific and social influences, a multitude of factors (McCormack, 1982) was discussed, which can lead to the cervical intraepithelial neoplasia (CIN). The two most important, but controversial factors are: (1) the influence of herpes simplex viruses (HSV-2) or papilloma viruses (HPV-1-8, HPV-6) and sexual behavior (Zur Hausen, 1977; Mumford, 1978; Bettendorf and Heerklotz, 1983). It seems that premature, intensive sexual activity beginning in puberty, especially promiscuity, contributes essentially to the development of precancerous changes of the uterine cervix (Rotkin, 1967). Harris *et al.* (1980) and Dietl *et al.* (1981) postulated this thesis, based on their own investigations, that precancerous changes of the uterine cervix were induced by sexual transmission. It is assumed that the most important factor seems to be the promiscuity and less important premature sexual activity. Frequent changes of sexual partners, rejection of barrier methods of contraception (condom, diaphragm) and recurrent genital inflammations are characteristics of women with cervical intraepithelial neoplasia according to the investigations of Dietl *et al.* (1981). It is suspected that the local immunologic barrier of the vaginal milieu, which was induced by the antigens of a constant partner, are broken through by new sexual partners and cervical intraepithelial neoplasia can possibly be caused, based on inflammatory reactions. Through this assumption the phenomenon can be explained, and a connection between oral contraceptive use and induction of precancerous changes of the uterine cervix was discussed by many investigators (Guhr, 1965; Dallenbach-Hellweg *et al.*, 1971; Swan and Brown, 1981). In women using barrier methods of contraception a low rate of precancerous changes of the uterine cervix was seen in comparison to the non-users of barrier methods (e.g. users of oral contraceptives and intrauterine devices), who are relatively unprotected against sexually transmitted diseases, according to many authors. Barrier methods of contraception act as a prophylactic agent against cervical intraepithelial neoplasia according to Wright *et al.* (1978) and Richardson and Lyon (1981).

Investigations about the effects on cervical epithelia by the method of menstrual hygiene, especially after evaluation in combination with the method of contraception, have not been satisfactorily performed with the exception of general publications on the use and side-effects of tampons (Dickinson, 1945; Thomas, 1966). More attention was given in past years to the use of tampons for menstrual hygiene due to the rare toxic shock syndrome (TSS, less than $1^{0}/_{00}$ per year). Most of the presently used tampons have a 50-year history. After widespread use of the tampons, claims were made that they lead to multiple diseases, e.g. endometritis, endometriosis, vaginitis and others (Wheatley and Geiger, 1965). Many of these supposed suspicions have been refuted. It could be proved that neither a meaningful influence on vaginal bacteriology (Magid and Geiger, 1942; Brand, 1952) nor effects on cervical cytology took place (Rutherford *et al.*, 1962). No negative influences on erosions of the uterine cervix could be proven according to the investigations of Thornton (1943) and Wheatley *et al.* (1965). They demonstrated that neither indications for the induction of

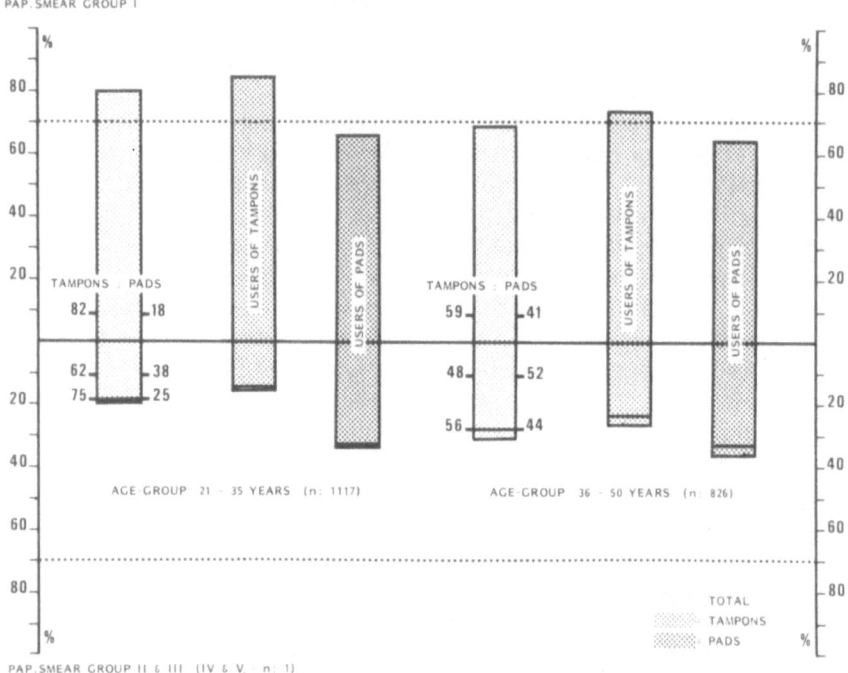

Figure 2.1 Cytological results (Munich Scheme, Pap smear groups I-V), menstrual hygiene (tampons or pads) and age-groups (21-35 and 36-50 years). $n = 1943$

neoplasia of the uterine cervix nor criteria for retrograde transuterine/transtubal discharge of cellular components including menstrual blood could be observed in a cohort of 2627 woman-years of use. In this investigation diseases induced by tampons were not found.

In a recent cytological investigation (Koch, 1982) with 1943 women, divided in age groups and methods of menstrual hygiene, the following results were gained within the framework of cancer detection screening (Figure 2.1): (1) the majority of younger women used tampons for menstrual hygiene, (2) there were no indications of an increased risk in tampon users for the induction of cervical intraepithelial neoplasia. The cytological Pap smears were evaluated and documented by the Munich scheme according to Soost and Baur (1980), and the tampon-using young women showed the largest proportion of Pap smear group I. In the group of older women the proportions of the Pap smear groups were less favorable. The distribution shows that the results of Pap smear group III (dubious) were three times higher. The results of Pap smear group II (atypical, unsuspicious) were also increased in the group using tampons (older women). In both age groups the pad users demonstrated the least favorable distribution in the cytological Pap smear group statistical analysis. It is difficult to explain this phenomenon. It is possible, that in the case of correct use of tampons, an inhibitory effect against infections is created due to the removal of the alkaline menstrual blood, which acts as a possible medium for the

28

growth of pathogenic bacteria and a buffer for the acidic vaginal milieu. This mechanism could explain the reduction of genital inflammations in tampon users as well as the more favorable distribution in the Pap smear groups; this distribution is related to the Pap smear groups I and II in combination with the various methods of menstrual hygiene. Other effects of the methods of menstrual hygiene, especially the induction of precancerous changes, could not be observed.

EFFECTS OF COPPER IUDs ON CERVICAL CYTOLOGY IN COMPARISON WITH OTHER METHODS OF CONTRACEPTION AND INFLUENCES OF COITAL FREQUENCY

Typical changes of the endometrium cannot be seen in users of barrier methods of contraception (condoms, diaphragms with spermicides). In contrast, specific changes of the endometrium are usually typical in the use of oral contraceptives as well as after insertion of IUDs. In addition, external influences on the endometrium and the uterine cervix, are possible by sexual behavior (frequency of cohabitation, promiscuity and others).

In addition to the above-mentioned foreign body reaction caused by the influence of IUDs, the specific effects of copper-bearing IUDs are the following: copper is able to affect the myometrial estrogen receptors (Lövgren et al., 1978), the estrogen uptake and the progesterone-binding capacity of the endometrium (Bonaventura et al., 1978). It also produces an interference with enzyme systems (Oster, 1972; Hagenfeldt, 1972), disturbances in glucose metabolism (Robles et al., 1972), an increase of the protein content of the endometrial fluid, an interference with cellular DNA and RNA (Hagenfeldt and Johannisson, 1972; Hagenfeldt, 1972; Mizumoto et al., 1976), as well as an inhibition of sperm motility and survival in the immediate period following insertion as described previously by us (Zielske et al., 1974).

The morphological findings in the endometrium with copper-bearing IUDs are demonstrated in Table 2.1.

Table 2.1 Morphological findings in women with copper-bearing IUDs

Endometrium histology	Endometrium cytology
Thinning of superficial epithelial cells	Loss of cilia and microvilli
Superficial ulcerations	Cytoplasm
Superficial lesions	vesiculation
Disturbances of re-epithelization	plasmolysis
Disturbances of cyclic development	Nucleus
Pseudodecidual stroma	enlargement
Edema of the stroma	vesiculation
Broadening of the capillaries	swelling
Lesions of the capillaries	prominent nucleoles
Inflammatory cells	alteration of chromatin
stroma	pseudo-eosinophilia
surface epithelium	
uterine fluid	
(Neutrophils, lymphocytes, plasma cells,	
macrophages)	

The reaction of the endometrium, which is caused by surface contact with the foreign body, shows a picture of a sterile reparable inflammation in the superficial layer of the endometrium which is eliminated during menstruation. Considerable disturbances of the endometrial proliferation and secretion phases were observed especially with the copper-bearing intrauterine devices in the immediate vicinity of this foreign body. On the one hand, there was a delayed development of the endometrium and on the other hand, insufficient thickening of the endometrial layer and a flattening of the epithelium. Furthermore, there were defects of the epithelium in the sense of small mucosal alterations with infiltration of leukocytes. In the framework of a study with the copper-bearing IUD ML Cu 250 (Koch and Vogel, 1980), biopsies were taken during different phases of the cycle and after different lengths of time of IUD use. Only some of the endometrial preparations were without the so-called mucosal inflammatory reaction; most of the preparations showed cellular extravasation of different intensity. Sometimes this reaction was very slight with only focal perivascular migration of a few granulocytes. There was also a diffuse subepithelial granulocytic migration which was also found in the middle layers. Remarkably, there were plaques of granulocytes, sometimes accompanied by lymphocytes, plasma cells and phagocytes. Often the superficial layer of the epithelium contained very well preserved granulocytes which were independent of the intensity of stromal reaction. In contrast to the superficial epithelium the glandular epithelium very rarely contained granulocytes and, if any, very few. This accompanying reaction consisted of an edema, which was rarely significant and showed only a slight broadening of the capillaries. Disturbances in the cyclic development of the mucosa were observed in 50% of all cases. On the one hand, retarded and reduced proliferation of the glands was seen, while on the other hand, there was insufficient secretory transformation with the beginning of desquamation.

Ultrastructural investigations of the endometrium, influenced by copper-bearing IUDs, have been performed by Nilsson and Hagenfeldt (1973), El-Badrawi et al. (1979) and Ludwig and Metzger (1976). There are specific endometrial changes near the copper wire. These changes of the epithelium are caused by the direct influence of the copper primarily, and secondarily there is an indirect influence of the copper ions on the metabolism of the epithelial cells.

The morphological changes of the endometrium, described above, can regularly be observed in the uterine cavity, where the IUD is located. The threads of the IUD are situated at the level of the uterine cervix and embedded in the cervical mucus; alterations of the endometrial cervical epithelia by mechanical influences occasionally may occur, but normally these effects are very slight due to the very small diameter of the monofil threads used. Only very small amounts of secretion from the endometrial uterine cavity together with cellular components reach the cervical canal. Most of the secretions of the uterine cavity, the cellular components included, were reabsorbed or phagocytized during the cycle with the exception of the menstrual phase due to the loss of the cervical mucus plug and the opening of the uterine cervix. Therefore, IUD-specific changes, which are typical for the uterine cavity, can only occasionally be found at the level of the uterine cervix. This confirms the experiences in cancer detection screenings, to diagnose an endometrial adenocarcinoma of the cavity by cervical Pap smears; normally only 10–20% of these carcinomas were detected by cervical smears (Reagan, 1973). On the other hand, it is possible that abnormal cells out of the uterine cavity, caused by the IUD, reach the uterine cervix. These cells often create difficulties in the diagnostic procedure, especially when the use of an IUD is unknown. Slight morphological changes of cervical epithelia can be caused by the threads of the IUD, e.g. microlesions of the external os, due directly to cohabitation can be observed and/or inflammatory reaction, due to the ascension of bacteria along the threads of the IUD. These reactions remain rare, due to the optimal immunological situation at the level of the uterine cervix (Schumacher, 1973). These results were confirmed by cytological investigations that will be discussed later in this chapter.

In observing atypical endometrial cells, especially in women over 40 years, although an IUD is in place, in differential cytological evaluation, the possibility of the presence of an endometrial adenocarcinoma must be considered (Fornari, 1974). In 1970, Ishihama et al. were able to prove in a large study ($n = 8284$; $n = 1058$ were IUD users) the carcinogenic risk in IUD users and a control group; they found no significant differences although false interpretations in IUD users cannot be ruled out, which can lead to an increase in the statistics of pathological Pap smears by methodical errors. With this and other comprehensive investigations (Richart and Barron, 1967), the apparent correlation between suspicious Pap smears and the use of IUDs established by Ayre (1965a, b) and Pincus (1965) could be refuted. Evidently, endometrial cells changed by the foreign body (caused by the IUD) were misinterpreted (Gupta et al., 1978). Richart and Barron (1967) emphasized that it is difficult to gain homogeneous cohorts for such investigations. Usually, an individually suited contraceptive method is recommended. Normally, in women with completed family planning, IUDs were inserted more frequently in comparison to nulliparous women. In addition, there is a correlation between increasing parity and an increasing rate of women with dysplasia of the uterine cervix, which also can increase the possibility of false interpretations. Also the statistical comparative evaluations of Pincus and Garcia (1964) have been passionately discussed in the past. Pincus postulated that the use of oral contraceptives (Oestrogen/progestogen) leads to a decrease of the proportion of smears with signs of dysplasia, in contrast to IUD users, and based this on the suppressive effects of progestogens on dysplasias of the uterine cervix. On the one hand, Guhr (1965), Dallenbach-Hellweg et al. (1971) and other investigators (review by Soost and Joswig-Priewe, 1978) described an increase of the carcinogenic risk due to the use of oral contraceptives (estrogen/progestogen), on the other hand the majority of the cytological investigators (Soost et al., 1967; review by Soost and Joswig-Priewe, 1978; Rinehart and Felt, 1977; Knab, 1977; Moghissi, 1979) claim that there is no significant evidence for an increased carcinogenic risk in users of oral contraceptives. Kindermann (1973) and Wilkinson et al. (1976) maintain, based on histological investiga-

31

tions, that there is no evidence for the hypothesis of an induction of pre-cancerous or cancerous changes of the uterine cervix by oral contraceptives, as they are almost always accompanied with local inflammation of the uterine cervix. This is also in agreement with the results of other investigators (Wied *et al.*, 1966). It is very difficult to answer the question, whether a different contraceptive regimen acts as an inductive factor for cancer. Only by statistical evaluations with an extremely large cohort of women with comparative groups of age, sexual activity, age of first pregnancy, social status, race, intensity of medical control, cytological screenings included, can significant results be gained. Definite cohorts of women are inclined to use fixed methods of contraception (Pfleiderer, 1981) and the sexual behavior varies from one cohort to the other; these facts especially cause great difficulties in comparing homogeneous cohorts for statistical evaluations. It is not surprising that before the use of the selected method of contraception begins, significantly different rates of dysplasia were found in the groups of the selected contraceptive methods (prevalence rate). Melamed *et al.* (1969, 1973), Stern *et al.* (1970), and Dabances *et al.* (1974) found, for example, increased rates of dysplasia in women who chose the oral contraceptive regimen. Bibbo *et al.* (1971) demonstrated in women using oral contraceptives two-fold rates of dysplasia (2.31%) and three-fold rates (3.12%) in IUD users in comparison to women who used neither oral contraceptives nor IUDs. Also the proportion of carcinoma *in situ* was twice as high in the users of oral contraceptives and IUDs (0.57%). In contrast, the rates of carcinoma of the uterine cervix were the lowest in the women using oral contraceptives (0.04%), in comparison to the users of IUDs (0.11%) and the control group (0.14%). The lower rate of carcinoma of the uterine cervix in the group of oral contraceptive users was explained by Bibbo *et al.* as due to the more intensive cytological screening of these women. These results confirm those of Schrage (1965) and Wied *et al.* (1966). Significantly increasing incidence rates for neoplasias could not be demonstrated for any contraceptive method, when absolutely homogeneous cohorts were evaluated. In the composition of homogeneous cohorts, the sexual activity deserves a key position. False correlations between the use of different methods of contraception and the appearance of carcinoma of the uterine cervix can be found, when this factor is neglected. This could explain multiple contradictory analyses in this field as due to various methods of statistical evaluation (Boyce *et al.*, 1977; Meisels *et al.*, 1977). In a recent excellent study (Swan and Brown, 1981) women with carcinoma of the uterine cervix were statistically analyzed. It was primarily seen that there were positive correlations between sexual activity, the use of oral contraceptives and the appearance of carcinoma of the uterine cervix. But after preparing homogeneous cohorts with comparative sexual activity these investigators could no longer demonstrate a significant correlation between the use of oral contraceptives and the carcinoma of the uterine cervix. This confirms the hypothesis of Rotkin (1962, 1973), that increasing sexual activity (premature sexual intercourse, increased coital frequency, promiscuity) increases the possibility of developing a carcinoma of the uterine cervix, due to the probability of a sexually transmitted infection.

The herpes simplex viruses (Peltonen, 1965; Naib *et al.*, 1966; Nahmias *et al.*, 1970; Rawls *et al.*, 1970; Adam *et al.*, 1971; Catalano and Johnson, 1971; Petersen *et al.*, 1972; König *et al.*, 1975; Josey *et al.*, 1975; Thomas and Rawls, 1978; and others) and the papilloma viruses (Zur Hausen, 1977, 1981; Meisels, 1976, 1981; Meisels *et al.*, 1977a, b) have been discussed as inducing agents of cervical intraepithelial neoplasia (CIN). Women with cervical intraepithelial neoplasia or carcinoma of the uterine cervix often have significantly higher titers of herpes simplex virus antibodies. Also these women had more frequent herpes simplex infections in their medical history. But a causal relationship between herpes simplex infections and the changes of the uterine cervix, e.g. cervical intraepithelial neoplasia or carcinoma of the uterine cervix, cannot be significantly established (Petersen *et al.*, 1975; Zur Hausen, 1981; Pfleiderer, 1981). Also the importance of the papilloma viruses in the causal genesis of the carcinoma of the uterine cervix has not been satisfactorily proved (Zur Hausen, 1981). Intensive research is being done in the field of the viral genesis as well as the formal genesis of the cervical intraepithelial neoplasia (Pfleiderer, 1981).

Basically, two forms of growth of the cervical intraepithelial neoplasia and the carcinoma of the cervix can be differentiated. The importance of sexual transmission is accepted for the one type of carcinoma of the uterine cervix. On the one hand, a slow developing type of the carcinoma of the uterine cervix begins with the passage of the different phases of the cervical intraepithelial neoplasia (Barron *et al.*, 1978; Richart, 1968), on the other hand the fast developing type of carcinoma of the uterine cervix begins primarily without or with very quick passage of the CIN-phases. Therefore, in the latter cancer detection screening always comes too late.

With the knowledge that the causal genesis of carcinoma of the cervix is a multifactorial occurrence, and that sexually transmitted agents are of importance for the development of cervical intraepithelial neoplasia, various parameters in the above-mentioned cohort (Koch, 1982) were investigated in addition to the cytological evaluations, e.g. age, menstrual hygiene, contraceptive methods, vaginal microbes and leukocytosis, and coital frequency. The following results were cytologically evaluated according to the recommendations of Soost and Baur (1980, 'Munich Scheme'). In all contraception groups ($n = 1943$) (Figures 2.2 and 2.3) the tampon users of the younger women (21–35 years) had the largest proportion of inconspicuous cytological results (Pap smear group I). The proportion of Pap smear group I of the users of the IUD (ML Cu 250) amounted to 89.5%. This distribution was the most favorable of the whole study (Koch, 1982). Only the younger users of pads in combination with spermicides with barrier methods showed an exception in the most unfavorable Pap smear group distribution. The group of older women (36–50 years) showed comparable results. The comparison of the different methods of contraception in combination with the cytological results of cervical Pap smears and in addition to the species of microbes and the proportions of leukocytes showed (Figures 2.4 and 2.5), that the so-called pure Döderlein bacilli flora was only seen in every fourth woman. The majority of the investigated women presented a so-called bacterial mixed flora, and in 15% of these women

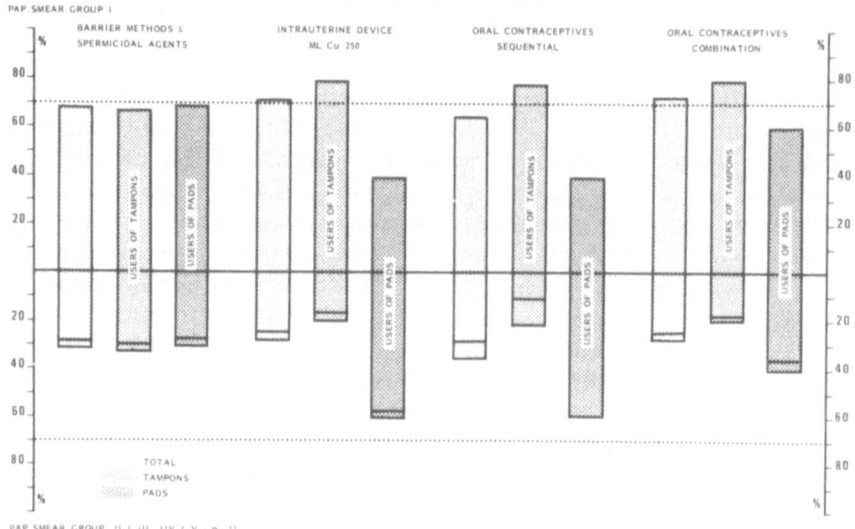

Figure 2.2 Cytological results (Munich Scheme, Pap smear groups I-V), menstrual hygiene (tampons or pads), contraception (barrier methods and spermicidal agents, IUD Ml Cu 250, oral contraceptives) and age-group (21-35 years). $n = 1117$

Candida albicans and/or *Trichomonas vaginalis* were observed. The proportion of *Haemophilus* (*gardnerella*) *vaginalis* in the group with the bacterial mixed flora amounted to 25%. For simplification of the figures only the group with Döderlein bacilli was contrasted to the combined bacterial mixed flora group. In the younger contraception group using spermicidal agents

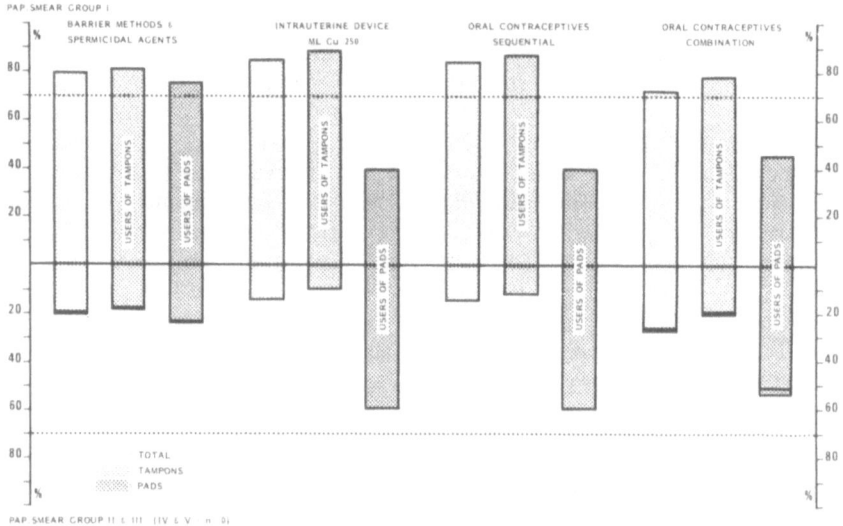

Figure 2.3 Cytological results (Munich Scheme, Pap smear groups I-V), menstrual hygiene (tampons or pads), contraception (barrier methods and spermicidal agents, IUD Ml Cu 250, oral contraceptives) and age-group (36-50 years). $n = 826$

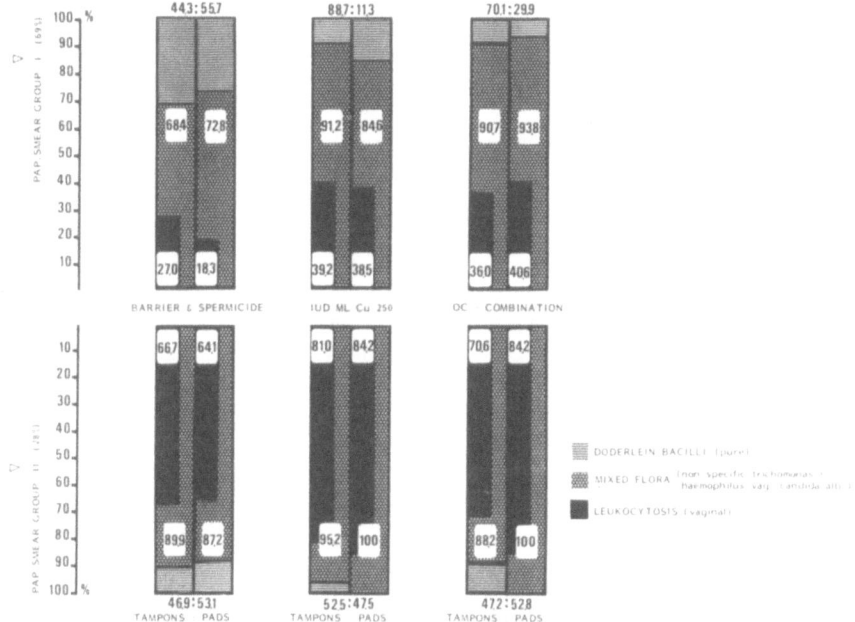

Figure 2.4 Cytological results (Munich Scheme, Pap smear groups I and II and vaginal micro-organisms), menstrual hygiene (tampons or pads), contraception (barrier methods and spermicidal agents, IUD ML Cu 250, oral contraceptives) and age-group (21-35 years). $n = 1117$

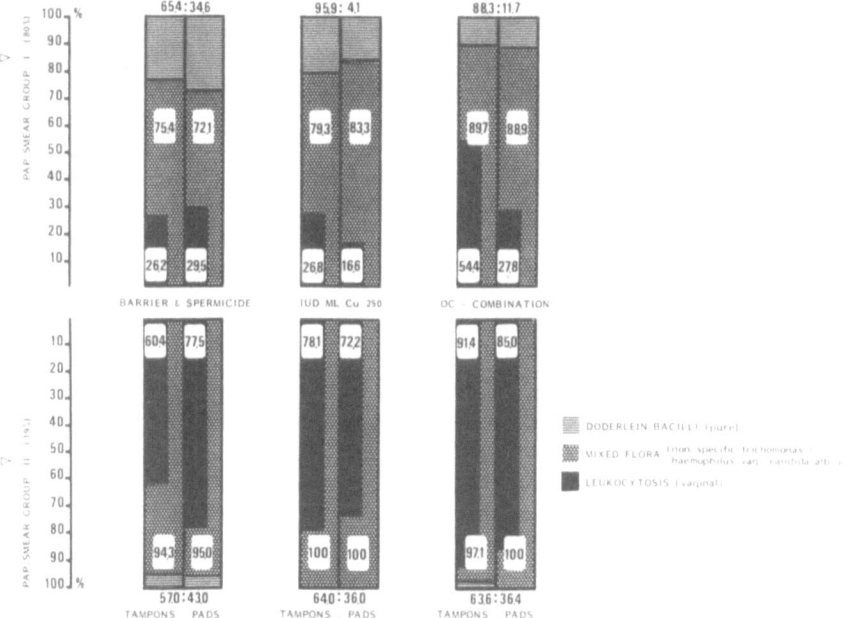

Figure 2.5 Cytological results (Munich Scheme, Pap smear groups I and II and vaginal micro-organisms), menstrual hygiene (tampons or pads), contraception (barrier methods and spermicidal agents, IUD ML Cu 250, oral contraceptives) and age-group (36-50 years). $n = 826$

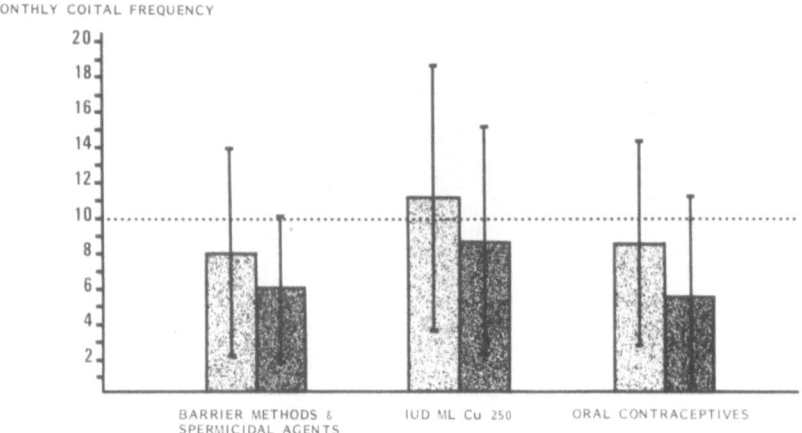

Figure 2.6 Monthly coital frequency, age-groups (21–35 and 36–50 years) and contraception (barrier methods with spermicidal agents, IUD ML Cu 250 and oral contraceptives). $n = 317$

with barrier methods, the users of pads with the Pap smear group I had the largest proportion of pure Döderlein bacilli flora (27.9%). The proportion of pure Döderlein bacilli flora was reduced in the group of women using oral contraceptives and of Pap smear group I; as was expected, in the Pap smear group II an almost total substitution of the pure Döderlein bacilli flora by the mixed bacterial flora took place; the proportion of vaginal leukocytosis was increased in Pap smear group II. Only in the Pap smear group I, in the younger women using oral contraceptives and tampons an increased proportion of vaginal leukocytosis was seen in 54.4%. The women with the IUD (ML Cu 250) and the women with spermicides with barrier methods did not differ in vaginal or cervical leukocytosis. In the age group of older women a similar status was seen; in the group of the women with the IUD (ML Cu 250) and Pap smear group I the proportion of pure Döderlein bacilli flora was reduced and the proportion with vaginal leukocytosis was increased in comparison to the younger women. The proportion of cervical leukocytosis amounted to only half of vaginal leukocytosis. It could be established that in IUD-bearing women there are no specific cytological changes at the level of the uterine cervix and that in these women the use of tampons could be recommended without hesitation.

The investigation of the influence of coital frequency in women using different methods of contraception (Figure 2.6) on the cytological results led to the following statistics: the mean monthly coital frequency was the highest in both age groups of IUD-bearing women. In the group of younger women with the IUD (ML Cu 250) *in situ* it amounted to 11.3 and in the older women to 8.6. The corresponding results in women using oral contraceptives were 8.5 and 5.5 and in women using spermicides with barrier methods 7.9 and 5.9. Although in IUD-bearing women no increase of cytopathological results could be observed and although these women showed the highest monthly coital frequency, it could be established that under these conditions an influence on the cervical cytology does not exist. These calculated data in this particular investigation do not lead to the conclusion that the contraceptive method influences the sexual activity, or that group specifically; women with different degrees of sexual activity prefer particular methods of contraception. The cytological data are in agreement with other investigators (Grumbrecht and Stoll, 1979; Stoll, 1981; Hilgarth, 1981).

Although in the area of the endometrial surface epithelium, which was in contact with the copper-bearing IUD, multiple IUD-specific cytological and histological changes can be seen (Moyer *et al.*, 1970, 1979; Herting and Tauber, 1978; Koch and Vogel, 1980), IUD-specific changes in the routine Pap smears of the uterine cervix cannot be expected. The method of menstrual hygiene (tampons or pads) did not show essential changes in the different groups of fertility regulation, especially in the group of IUD users; the use of tampons implies, when correctly used, no special risk. In our cohort of investigated women (Koch, 1982) no toxic shock syndrome was observed. It should be emphasized that the pad users had a higher proportion of Pap smear group II in most of the contraception and in all age groups. A special carcinogenic risk for the IUD users cannot be established, which is in accordance with most of the investigators (Tatum, 1981; Prinz *et al.*, 1981). The more frequent leukocytosis at the area of the vagina and the uterine cervix, without any clinical symptoms in users of the IUDs as well as oral contraceptives, has no pathological value and is meaningless.

EFFECTS OF COPPER IUDs ON TRANSTUBAL SPERM MIGRATION

In the past many investigations on the physiology of sperm migration were performed (Koch, 1980), especially in the field of the interaction between the spermatozoa and the mucus of the uterine cervix. In sterility work-ups, it was seen that there are direct correlations between spermatozoal recovery rates in the peritoneal fluid around the day of ovulation and the prognosis for later pregnancies (Koch *et al.*, 1974, 1977). In cases of fertile ejaculate and normal female genital tract and function, after cohabitation around the day of ovulation, in 50% of the investigated women spermatozoa could be detected in the peritoneal fluid after a single investigation. The highest spermatozoal recovery rate in the peritoneal fluid was found after intracavital AIH (0.1–0.2 ml ejaculate). The pregnancy rate was the highest in this cohort. In cases of patent Fallopian tubes and negative spermatozoal findings after intracavital AIH, pregnancies cannot be expected. An inhibition of the spermatozoal penetration at the level of the uterine cervix could be demonstrated in women using the IUD ML Cu 250 by *in vitro* and *in vivo* spermatozoal migration tests. In 50 women with the IUD ML Cu 250 *in situ* the sperm migration was investigated in the whole female genital tract (PSM Test: Peritoneal Sperm Migration Test, Koch *et al.*, 1974). Although in these women the postcoital tests according to Sims (1866) and Hühner (1913) around the day of ovulation were positive, no spermatozoa could be

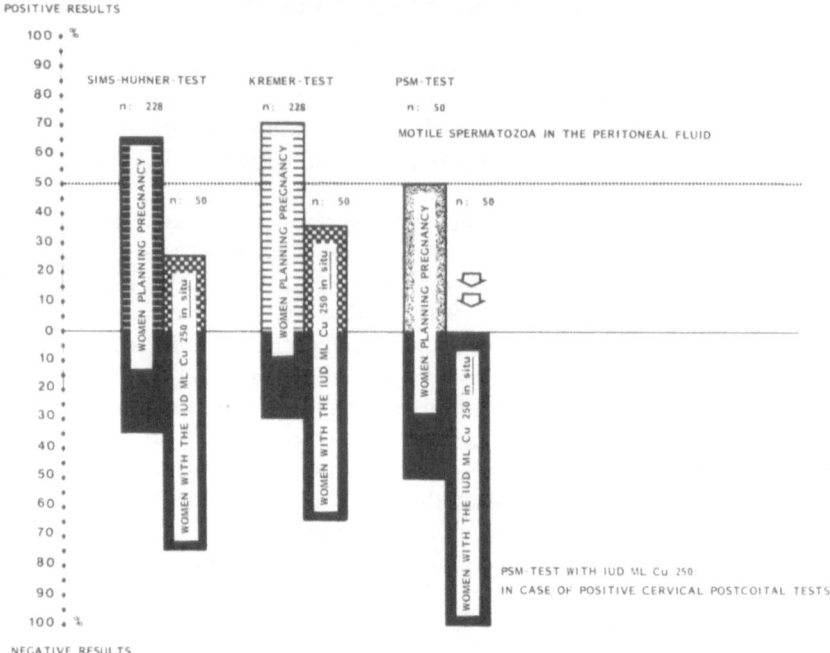

Figure 2.7 Postcoital test (according to Sims-Hühner), sperm migration test (according to Kremer) and peritoneal sperm migration test (PSM-test according to Koch, Hammerstein and Zielske) without and with the copper-bearing IUD ML Cu 250 *in situ*

detected in the peritoneal fluid (Figure 2.7). The differential cytological investigation of the secretions of the uterine cavity (Koch and Vogel, 1981) showed an increase of polymorphonuclear leukocytes and macrophages. Occasionally in the fluid of the uterine cavity, spermatozoa were observed, but most of them were without motility. The differential cytological investigation of the peritoneal fluid in women using the IUD (ML Cu 250) showed no significant abnormalities in comparison to the women with the desire for pregnancy. These results were in accordance with other investigators (Bercovici and Gallily, 1978). The ratio of macrophages with mesothelial cells, lymphocytes and polymorphonuclear leukocytes amounted in women with sterility 75:19:6% in the case of positive spermatozoal recovery in the peritoneal fluid and 80:16:4% in the case of negative spermatozoal findings. In 9 IUD ML Cu 250-bearing women, all with negative spermatozoal findings, the ratio was 69:17:14%.

The elimination of spermatozoa takes place in the entire female genital tract by macrophages and polymorphonuclear leukocytes (Hafez, 1973, 1978; Koch and Vogel, 1981). An increased proportion of leukocytes in the cervical mucus in combination with normal cervical factors does not disturb sperm migration, due to the micellar ultrastructure of the cervical mucus which protects the spermatozoa against phagocytosis. This phenomenon is only observed at the level of the uterine cervix. Phagocytosis of spermatozoa by macrophages and other leukocytes is improved in the uterine cavity, the oviducts and the abdominal cavity. The foreign body reaction, caused by the IUD, produces a local leukocytosis in the fluids of the uterine cavity as well as in the oviducts, the media for sperm migration (Beerthuizen *et al.*, 1979; Eschenbach and Soderstrom, 1979). The direct cell contact between spermatozoa and phagocytes, especially macrophages, is made possible by the increased count of polymorphonuclear leukocytes and macrophages in the secretions of the capillary spaces of the upper female genital tract (uterine cavity, oviducts), if there is an IUD in place (Koch and Vogel, 1981). A partial effect in the multifactorial mode of action of the copper-bearing IUDs seems to be the inhibition of transtubal sperm migration, which is a parameter of fertility according to our previous results (Koch *et al.*, 1974), due to an increased spermatozoal elimination by the increased counts of leukocytes. The endometrial foreign body reaction, caused by the IUD, inhibits or blocks the transtubal sperm migration due to the increased spermatozoal phagocytosis. Tubal spermatozoa were found when inert IUDs were inserted (Mastroianni and Honsanand, 1964; Malkani and Sujan, 1964; Morgenstern *et al.*, 1966) and Croxatto *et al.* (1975) observed in five out of seven cases tubal spermatozoa in IUD Cu T 200 users and in one case spermatozoa in the peritoneal cavity.

On the one hand, it could be demonstrated that in every second woman with the desire for pregnancy and with normal female genital tract and function positive spermatozoal recovery rates in the peritoneal fluid at midcycle can be expected, and, on the other hand, in spite of positive postcoital cervical sperm migration tests, no spermatozoa were detected in the peritoneal fluid in women with the IUD ML Cu 250 *in situ*. These results could establish, that in women with the IUD (ML Cu 250) the endometrial leukocytosis with increased phagocytosis of spermatozoa seems to be an important factor in the IUD's multifactorial mode of action. The large proportion of macrophages in the uterine fluid in IUD users with increased spermatozoal phagocytosis, as described by Sagiroglu and Sagiroglu (1970), was confirmed. The influences on the blastocyst according to Sagiroglu and Sagiroglu (1970) are of minor importance in the mode of IUD's action, because, according to the demonstrated results (Koch, 1982) in cases of disturbed sperm migration, a fertilization does not normally occur.

CONCLUDING REMARKS

Only inadequate answers to the multiple problems, discussed in this chapter, were possible by referring to personally collected data and those of other investigators. In conclusion, it can be established that there is no evidence for the induction of precancerous or cancerous changes of the uterine cervix due to the use of IUDs or other contraceptive methods. We know that women with fixed methods of contraception belong to definite cohorts with different sexual activity. In the statistical evaluation of the cytological results and the use of different methods of menstrual hygiene there were no significant signs for a negative influence on the epithelia of the uterine cervix due to the use of tampons. Pad users showed more often less favorable Pap smears. It is not necessary to give any recommendations for the use of a special method of menstrual hygiene in the different contraception groups. The risk of getting a vaginal infection is increased, as expected, in the cohort of women not using barrier methods of contraception, especially in women over 35 years. The inhibition of transtubal sperm migration in the users of the IUD ML Cu 250 seems to be the most important factor in the multifactorial mode of action. Therefore, the possible inhibition of implantation of the blastocyst is unimportant when fertilization does not normally occur.

References

Adam, E., Levy. A. H., Rawls, W. E. and Melnick, I. L. (1971). Seroepidemiologic studies of herpes-virus type 2 and carcinoma of the cervix. I. Case-control. *J. Natl. Cancer Inst.*, **47**, 941

Ayre, J. E. (1965a). Human precarcinogenic cell manifestations associated with polyethylene contraceptive device. *Indust. Med. Surg.*, **34**, 393

Ayre, J. E. (1965b). Vaginal smear studies on IUD. *Indust. Med. Surg.*, **34**, 993

Barron, B. A., Cahill, M. C. and Richart, R. M. (1978). A statistical model of the material history of cervical neoplastic disease: the duration of carcinoma *in situ*. *Gynecol. Oncol.*, **6**, 196

Beerthuizen, R. J. C. M., van Wijk, J. A. M., Eskes, T. K. A. B., Vermeulen, A. H. M. and Vooijs, G. P. (1979). Pathomorphologic changes in the oviducts in IUD patient. In *Proceedings International Symposium, Medicated IUDs and Polymeric Delivery Systems*, Amsterdam

Bercovici, B. and Gallily, R. (1978). The cytology of the human peritoneal fluid. *Acta Cytologica*, **22**, 124

Bettendorf. U. and Heerklotz, D. (1983). Virusinfektionen der Cervix uteri: Herpes simplex genitalis und Condylomata acuminata. *Deut. Ärzteblatt*, **80**, 27

Bibbo, M., Keebler, C. M. and Wied, G. L. (1971). Prevalence and incidence rates of cervical atypia. A computerized file analysis of 148735 patients. *J. Reprod. Med.*, **6**, 184

Bonaventura, L. M., Creary, R. E. and Young, P. C. M. (1978). The *in vivo* effects of copper on specific progesterone binding by human endometrium cytosol. *Fertil. Steril.*, *Suppl.*, **30**, 741

Boyce, J. G., Lu, T., Nelson, J. H. and Fruchter, R. G. (1977). Oral contraceptives and cervical carcinoma. *Am. J. Obstet. Gynecol.*, **128**, 761

Boyes, D. A. (1975). Age for routine cervical Papanicolaou screening tests. *J. Am. Med. Assoc.*, **232**, 961

Brand, E. (1952). Bacteriology and vaginal flora after use of internal tampons. *Br. Med. J.*, **1**, 24

Catalano, L. W. Jr. and Johnson, L. D. (1971). Herpes virus antibody and carcinoma *in situ* of the cervix. *J. Am. Med. Assoc.*, **217**, 447

Croxatto, H. B., Faundes, A., Medel. M., Avendano, S., Croxatto, H. D., Vera, C., Anselmo, J. and Pastene, L. (1975). Studies on sperm migration in the human female genital tract. In Hafez, E. S. E. and Thibault, C. G. (eds) *The Biology of Spermatozoa. INSERM International Symposium*, pp. 56 62 Nouzilly. (Basel: Karger)

Dabances, A., Prado, R., Larraguibel, P. and Zanartu, J. (1974). Intraepithelial cervical neoplasia in women using intrauterine devices and long-acting injectable progestogens as contraceptives. *Am. J. Obstet. Gynecol.*, **116**, 1052

Dallenbach-Hellweg, G., Herting, W., Momber, F. and Thorn, V. (1971). Zytologische und histologische Untersuchungen der Portio und Cervix uteri unter der Einnahme von Ovulationshemmern. *Fortschr. Med.*, **89**, 883

Dickinson, R. L. (1945). Tampons as menstrual guard. *J. Am. Med. Assoc.*, **128**, 490

Dietl, J., Buchholz, F. and Semm, K. (1981). Zur epidemiologie und Diagnostik der Vor- und Frühformen des Collum-Carcinoms. *Geburtsh. Frauenheilkd.*, **41**, 173

El-Badrawi, H., Hafez, E. S. E., Makebe, S. and van Os, W. A. A. (1979). S.E.M. of human endometrium with ML Cu-250 or inert IUD. In *Proceedings of International Symposium, Medicated IUDs and Polymeric Delivery Systems*, Amsterdam

Eschenbach, D. A. and Soderstrom, R. M. (1979). IUD and salpingitis. In *Proceedings of International Symposium, Medicated IUDs and Polymeric Delivery Systems*, Amsterdam

Fornari, M. L. (1974). Cellular changes in the glandular epithelium of patients using IUCD - a source of cytologic error. *Acta Cytologica*, **18**, 341

Grumbrecht, C. and Stoll, P. (1979). Zytologische Veränderungen bei IUD-Trägerinnen. Presented at the *5th Fortbildungstagung für klinische Zytologie*, München

Guhr, O. (1965). Kolposkopische, zytologische und histologische Portiobefunde bei ovulationshemmenden Medikamenten. *Arch. Gynäk.*, **202**, 205

Gupta, P. K., Burroughs, F., Luff, R. D., Frost, J. K. and Erozan, Y. S. (1978). Epithelial atypias associated with intrauterine contraceptive devices (IUD). *Acta Cytologica*, **22**, 286

Hafez, E. S. E. (1973). *Human Reproduction*. (Hagerstown: Harper & Row)

Hafez, E. S. E. (1978). Transport and survival of spermatozoa in the human female reproductive tract. In Ludwig, H. and Tauber, P. F. (eds) *Human Fertilization*, pp. 119-127. (Stuttgart: Thieme)

Hagenfeldt, K. (1972). Intrauterine contraception with the copper-T device. *Contraception*, **6**, 37, 191, 207, 219

Hagenfeldt, K. and Johannisson, E. (1972). The effect of intrauterine copper on DNA content in the isolated human endometrial cells. *Acta Cytologica*, **16**, 472

Harris, R. W. C., Brinton, L. A., Cowdell, R. H., Skegg, D. C. G., Smith, P. G., Vessey, M. P. and Doll, R. (1980). Characteristics of women with dysplasia or carcinoma *in situ* of the cervix uteri. *Br. J. Cancer*, **42**, 359

Herting, W. and Tauber, P. F. (1978). Endometrium-Zytologie bei kupferhaltigen Intrauterinpessaren. *Fortschr. Med.*, **96**, 311

Hilgarth, M. (1981). Zytologische Veränderungen bei Trägerinnen von Kupfer-Pessaren. Presented at *IUD-Symposium*, Helsinki/Kiel

Hühner, M. (1913). *Sterility in the Male and Female and its Treatment*. (New York: Rebman Co.)

Ishihama, A., Kagatu, T., Imai, T. and Shima, M. (1970). Cytologic studies after insertion of intrauterine contraceptive devices. *Acta Cytologica*, **14**, 35

Josey, W. E., Nahmias, A. J. and Naib, Z. M. (1975). Der augenblickliche Stand der Herpesvirus-Zervixkarzinom-Theorie. *Geburtsh. Frauenheilkd.*, **35**, 425

Kindermann, G. (1973). Beeinflussung des Zervixepithels durch Ovulationshemmer aus der Sicht des Klinikers und Morphologen. *Mitt.-Dienst Ges. Bekämpf. Krebskrh. Nordrhein-Westfalen*, **4**, 839

Knab, D. R. (1977). Estrogen and endometrial carcinoma. *Obstet. Gynecol. Surv.*, **32**, 267

Koch, U. J. (1980). Sperm migration in the human female genital tract with and without intrauterine devices. *Acta Europaea Fertilitatis*, **11**, 733

Koch, U. J. (1982). Klinisch-zytologischer Erfahrungsbericht über das IUD ML Cu 250. In *Die intrauterine Kontrazeption. Fortschritte der Fertilitätsforschung*, **10**, 71 (Berlin: Grosse)

Koch, U. J., Hammerstein, J. and Zielske, F. (1977). Clinical meaning of spermatozoa found in the peritoneal fluid after vaginal and intrauterine insemination. *Fertil. Steril.*, **28**, 310

Koch, U. J. and Vogel, M. (1980). Effects of ML Cu 250 on the endometrium and sperm migration together with clinical results. *Contracept. Deliv. Syst.*, **1**, 37

Koch, U. J. and Vogel, M. (1981). Leukocytes and their influence on sperm migration in the human female genital tract including the peritoneal cavity. In Semm, K. and Mettler, L. (eds) *Proceedings of the 3rd World Congress, Human Reproduction*, pp. 501-506. (Amsterdam: Excerpta Medica)

Koch, U. J., Zielske, F. and Hammerstein, J. (1974). Nachweis der Spermatozoenaszension im weiblichen Genitaltrakt als Routineuntersuchung in der Sterilitätsdiagnostik. *Arch. Gynäk.*, **219**, 610

Köng, U. D., Haag, A., Lehmköster, A. and Schneweis, K. E. (1975). Seroepidemiologische Untersuchungen zur Frage des Kausalzusammenhangs zwischen der Herpes-genitalis-Infektion und der Entstehung des Kollum-Karzinoms. *Geburtsh. Frauenheilkd.*, **35**, 909

Lövgren, T., Pettersson, K., Lundberg, B. and Punnonen, R. (1978). Effect of Cu^{2+} ions on the binding of estrogen to the human myometrial estrogen binding protein. *Contraception*, **18**, 181

Ludwig, H. and Metzger, H. (1976). *The Human Female Reproductive Tract*. (Berlin-Heidelberg-New York: Springer)

McCormack, W. M. (1982). Sexually transmitted diseases: women as victims. *J. Am. Med. Assoc.*, **248**, 177

Magid, M. O. and Geiger, J. (1942). The intravaginal tampon in menstrual hygiene. A clinical study. *Med. Rec.*, (cited by Thomas (1966))

Malkani, P.K. and Sujan, S. (1964). Sperm migration in the female reproductive tract in the presence of intrauterine devices. *Am. J. Obstet. Gynecol.*, **88**, 934

Mastroianni, L. and Honsanand, C. (1964). Intrauterine contraception. In *Proceedings of the 2nd International Conference*. (Amsterdam: Excerpta Medica)

Meisels, A., Begin, R. and Schneider, V. (1977, p. 194). Dysplasias of the uterine cervix. Epidemiological aspects: role of age at first coitus and use of oral contraceptives. *Cancer*, **40**, 3076

Meisels, A. (1976). Condylomatous lesions of the cervix and vagina. I. Cytologic patterns. *Acta Cytol.*, **20**, 505

Meisels, A., Fortin, R. and Roy, M. (1977b). Condylomatous lesions of the cervix. II. Cytologic, colposcopic and histopathologic study. *Acta Cytol.*, **21**, 379

Meisels, A. (1981). Klinisch-diagnostische Bezüge zur Virusinfektion. Vortrag III. *Int. Tutorial über das diagnostische und therapeutische Vorgehen bei frühen zervikalen und intrauterinen Neoplasien*. Freiburg 4.4.1981

Melamed, M. R. and Flehinger, B. J. (1973). Early incidence rates of precancerous cervical lesions in women using contraceptives. *Gynecol. Oncol.*, **1**, 290

Melamed, M. R., Koss, L. G., Flehinger, B. J., Kelisky, R. P. and Dubrow, H. (1969). Prevalence rates of uterine cervical carcinoma *in situ* for women using diaphragm or contraceptive oral steroids. *Br. Med. J.*, **3**, 195

Mizumoto, H., Hohman, W. R. and Moyer, D. L. (1976). Effects of IUDs on DNA metabolism in rabbit blastocysts. *Fertil. Steril.*, **27**, 449

Moghissi, K. S. (1977). Oral contraceptives and endometrial and cervical cancer. *J. Toxicol. Environ. Health*, **3**, 243

Morgenstern, L. L., Orgebin-Crist, M-C., Clewe, T. H., Bonney, W. A. and Noyes, R. W. (1966). Observations on spermatozoa in the human uterus and oviducts in the chronic presence of intrauterine devices. *Am. J. Obstet. Gynecol.*, **96**, 114

Moyer, D. L., El-Sahwi, S., Macaulay, L. and Shaw, S. T. (1979). Cells of the uterine fluid. In Beller, F. K. and Schumacher, G. F. B. (eds) *The Biology of the Fluids of the Female Genital Tract*, pp. 59–72. (New York: Elsevier)

Moyer, D. L., Mishell, D. R. and Bell, J. (1970). Reactions of human endometrium to the intrauterine device. *Am. J. Obstet. Gynecol.*, **106**, 799

Moyer, D. L. and Shaw, S. T. (1980). Mode of action of intrauterine devices. In: Human Reproduction, p. 661–681, editor: E. S. E. Hafez (Hagerstown: Harper & Row).

Mumford, D. M. (1978). Immunity of herpes simplex virus and cervical carcinoma. *Surg. Clin. N. Am.*, **58**, 39

Myatt, L., Chaudhuri, G., Gordon, D. and Elder, M. G. (1977). Prostaglandin production by leukocytes attached to intrauterine devices. *Contraception*, **15**, 589

Nahmias, A. J., Josey, W. E., Naib, Z. M., Luce, C. F. and Guest, B. A. (1970). Antibodies to herpes-virus hominis types 1 and 2 in humans. II. Women with cervical cancer. *Am. J. Epidemiol.*, **91**, 547

Naib, Z. M., Nahmias, A. J. and Josey, W. E. (1966). Cytology and histopathology of cervical herpes simplex infection. *Cancer*, **19**, 1026

Nilsson, O. and Hagenfeldt, K. (1973). Scanning electron microscopy of human uterine epithelium influenced by the T Cu intrauterine contraceptive device. *Am. J. Obstet. Gynecol.*, **117**, 469

Oster, G. K. (1972). Chemical reactions of the copper intrauterine device. *Fertil. Steril.*, **23**, 18

Peltonen, R. (1965). Antibodies to herpes-virus hominis types 1 and 2 among women with neoplastic change of uterine cervix. *Acta Obstet. Gynecol. Scand.*, **54**, 369

Petersen, E. E., Böcker, J. F., Fürmaier, I. and Hillemanns, H. G. (1972). Herpes simplex virus Typ 2: Seine Verbreitung und seine Beziehung zum Zervixkarzinom. *Dtsch. Med. Wochenschr.*, **97**, 1936

Petersen, E. E., Böcker, J. F., Schmitt, M., Wimhöfer, G. and Hillemanns, H. G. (1975). Zervixkarzinom und Herpes-simplex-virus Typ 2. Untersuchungen zur Frage eines Kausalzusammenhanges. *Geburtsh. Frauenheilkd.*, **35**, 98

Pfleiderer, A. (1981). Entwicklungsgeschichte der cervikalen, intraepithelialen Neoplasie. *Gynäkologe*, **14**, 194

Pincus, G. (1965). Intrauterine contraception. In *Proceedings of 2nd International Conference.* p. 207. Int. Congress Series 86. (Amsterdam: Excerpta Medica)

Pincus, G. and Garcia, C. R. (1964). Preliminary findings on hormonal steroids and vaginal, cervical and endometrial histology. *Revista Inst. Nac. Cancer (Mex.)*, **16**, 452

Prinz, W., Noack, J., Kraus, H. and Schuhmann, R. A. (1981). Zytologische Befunde beim Intrauterinpessar. *Geburtsh. Frauenheilkd.*, **41**, 194

Rawls, W. E., Gardner, H. L. and Kaufmann, R. L. (1970). Antibodies to herpes virus in patients with carcinoma of the cervix. *Am. J. Obstet. Gynecol.*, **108**, 710

Reagan, J. W. (1973). *The Cells of Uterine Adenocarcinoma.* (Basel: Karger)

Richardson, A. C. and Lyon, J. B. (1981). The effect of condom use on squamous cell cervical intraepithelial neoplasia. *Am. J. Obstet. Gynecol.*, **140**, 909

Richart, R. M. (1968). Natural history of cervical intraepithelial neoplasia. *Clin. Obstet. Gynecol.*, **10**, 748

Richart, R. M. and Barron, B. A. (1967). The intrauterine device and cervical neoplasia. *J. Am. Med. Assoc.*, **199**, 817

Rinehart, W. and Felt, J. C. (1977). *Oral Contraceptives.* Population Reports. Series A, No. 4. (Washington, DC: The George Washington University Medical Center)

Robles, F., Lopez de la Osa, E., Lerner, U., Johannisson, E., Brenner, P., Hagenfeldt, K. and Diczfalusy, E. (1972). Alpha-amylase, glycogen synthetase and phosphorylase in the human endometrium: influence of the cycle and of the Cu-T device. *Contraception*, **6**, 373

Rotkin, I. D. (1962). Relation of adolescent coitus to cervical cancer risk. *J. Am. Med. Assoc.* **179**, 486

Rotkin, I. D. (1967). Adolescent coitus and cervical cancer: associations of related events with increased risk. *Cancer Res.*, **27**, 603

Rotkin, I. D. (1973). A comparison review of key epidemiological studies in cervical cancer related to current searches for transmissible agents. *Cancer Res.*, **33**, 1353

Rutherford, R. N., Banks, A. L. and Coburn, W. A. (1962). Intravaginal tampons for the postpartum patient. *Obstet. Gynecol.*, **19**, 781

Sagiroglu, N. and Sagiroglu, E. (1970). The cytology of intrauterine contraceptive devices. *Acta Cytologica (Baltimore)*, **14**, 58

Schmidt-Elmendorff, H. R. and Eilemann, H. O. (1951). Clinical studies on intra-vaginal tampons as menstrual protection. *Zbl. Gynaek.*, **73**, 1507

Schrage, R. (1965). Die Zusammensetzung der weiblichen Klientel bei Krebsfrüherkennungsuntersuchungen. *Frauenarzt*, **4**, 266

Schumacher, G. F. B. (1973). Soluble proteins of human cervical mucus. In Elstein, M., Moghissi, K. and Borth, R. (eds) *Cervical Mucus in Human Reproduction. WHO Colloquium, Geneva*, pp. 93–113. (Copenhagen: Scriptor)

Sims, J. M. (1866). *Clinical Notes on Uterine Surgery.* (New York: W. Wood)

Soost, H. J. and Baur, S. (1980). *Gynaekologische Zytodiagnostik.* (Stuttgart, New York: George Thieme)

Soost, H. J. and Bayer, E. (1967). Einfluss der Ovulationshemmer auf das Gebaermutterhalsepithel. *Dtsch. Med. Wochenschr.*, **92**, 1789

Soost, H. J. and Joswig-Priewe, H. (1978). Einfluss oraler Ovulationshemmer auf die Kanzerogenese des Zervixepithels. *Arch. Geschwulstforsch.*, **48**, 345

Stern, E., Clark, H. A. and Coffelt, C. F. (1970). Contraceptives and dysplasia: higher rate for pill choosers. *Science*, **169**, 497

Stoll, P. (1981). Histologische und zytologische Befunde bei IUD-Trägerinnen. Presented at the *IUD Symposium*, Helsinki/Kiel

Swan, S. H. and Brown, W. L. (1981). Oral contraceptive use, sexual activity and cervical carcinoma. *Am. J. Obstet. Gynecol.*, **139**, 52

Tatum, H. J. (1981). Gegenwart und Zukunft der intrauterinen Kontrazeptiva. Presented at the *4th Int. Münsteraner Gespräch*

Thomas, C. L. (1966). The influence of menstrual protection devices on vaginal physiology. *J. Am. Coll. Health Assoc.*, **15**, 136

Thomas, D. B. and Rawls, W. E. (1978). Relationship of herpes simplex virus type 2 antibodies and squamous dysplasia to cervical carcinoma *in situ*. *Cancer*, **42**, 2716

Thornton, M. J. (1943). The use of vaginal tampons for the absorption of menstrual discharges. *Am. J. Obstet. Gynecol.*, **46**, 259

Wheatley, R. E., Menkin, M. F., Bardes, E. D. and Rock, J. (1965). Tampons in menstrual hygiene. *J. Am. Med. Assoc.*, **192**, 697

WHO Technical Report Series 619. (1978). *Steroid Contraception and the Risk of Neoplasia.* Report of a WHO Scientific Group, Geneva

Wied, G. L., Davis, E., Frank, R., Segal, P. B., Meier, P. and Rosenthal, D. (1966). Statistical evaluation of the effect of hormonal contraceptives in the appearance of the cytological smear pattern. *Obstet. Gynecol.*, **27**, 327

Wilkinson, E., Fazog, M. D. and Dufour, D. R. (1976). Pathogenesis of microglandular hyperplasia of the cervix uteri. *Obstet. Gynecol.*, **47**, 189

Wright, N. H., Vessey, M. P., Kenward, B., McPherson, K. and Doll, R. (1978). Neoplasia and dysplasia of the cervix uteri and contraception: a possible protective effect of the diaphragm. *Br. J. Cancer*, **38**, 273

Zielske, F., Koch, U. J., Badura, R. and Ladeburg, H. (1974). Studies on copper release from copper-T devices (T-Cu 200) and its influence on sperm migration *in vitro*. *Contraception*, **10**, 651

Zur Hausen, H. (1977). Human papillomaviruses and their possible role in squamous cell carcinomas. In *Current Topics in Microbiology and Immunology*. Vol 78. (Berlin, Heidelberg, New York: Springer)

Zur Hausen, H. (1981). Die Rolle der Virusinfektion bei der Karzinogenese der weiblichen Genitalkarzinome. Vortag. III. *Int. Tutorial über das diagnostische und therapeutische Vorgehen bei frühen zervikalen und intrauterinen Neoplasien*, Freiburg

3
Inflammatory changes induced by IUDs in animal models

P.K. MEHROTRA and K. SRIVASTAVA

Reports of inflammatory reaction in uterine endometrium in the presence of an IUD have been unequivocal (Greenwald, 1965; Parr, 1969; Parr and Segal, 1966; Williams and Peck, 1977). An inflammatory reaction appears to be a common denominator in almost every animal: mouse (Doyle and Margolis, 1965; Parr and Segal, 1966); hamster (Saksena et al., 1974); goat (Janakiraman et al., 1970); cow (Hawk et al., 1968); pig (Gerrits et al., 1968); rabbit (Ledger and Bickley, 1966); and sheep (Hawk, 1967), and leads to infiltration of numerous polymorphonuclear leukocytes, mononuclear cells and macrophages in the endometrium and uterine lumen (El Sahwi and Moyer, 1971; Parr and Segal, 1966). These cells possibly release some embryotoxic material in the uterine lumen (El Sahwi and Moyer, 1971; Parr, 1969, 1970).

This chapter considers possible factors involved in IUD-induced inflammatory changes in the uterus of different animals.

FACTORS INVOLVED IN IUD-INDUCED INFLAMMATION

Mechanical injury

The IUD is reported to cause a foreign body stress to the uterine endometrium, thereby interfering with its normal functioning. Such stress may also produce a traumatic effect on the vascular network of the uterus (Kar and Chandra, 1965, 1967), as a result of which stromal and epithelial cell differentiation is profoundly altered (Joshi and Gunn, 1971). Tissue injury leads to inflammation of which one of the cardinal signs is accumulation of leukocytes at the site (Bainton, 1980), a phenomenon noted with IUDs.

Cellular inflammation

Inflammation is known to provoke proliferation and multiplication of connective tissue cells; the extent and duration of this proliferative process is determined by the degree of cell injury or subsequent leukocytic exudation, or both (Dumont, 1965). The IUD also is reported to produce uterine hypertrophy in many species (Chaudhuri, 1971, 1973; Lau et al., 1974; Parr and Segal, 1966; Saksena et al., 1974; Williams and Peck, 1977), hyperplasia (Martin and Finn, 1979) and squamous metaplasia (Srivastava and Mehrotra, 1978) in lumenal epithelia of ovariectomized mice and normal rats, respectively. These uterine changes are possibly analogous to those appearing in other tissues as a consequence of inflammation.

Nucleoli in luminal epithelial cells of rat uterus are reported to appear and increase in size following IUD insertion (Parr, 1969). Since nucleoli are indicative of enhanced metabolic turnover of the cell, their appearance may reflect the augmentation of the cellular synthetic activity resulting in the proliferation of epithelial cells. Parr (1969) has associated this phenomenon with inflammation.

Proinflammatory changes—release of prostaglandins

Uterine distention or any alteration in uterine tissue components caused by an IUD may affect the vascular network of the endometrium, as a result of which proinflammatory prostaglandins, prostacyclin (PGI_2), are released (Shaw, 1980). The IUD also stimulates the production and/or release of certain other prostaglandins, such as PGE_2 and $PGF_{2\alpha}$ in uterine endometrium (Saksena et al., 1974). These prostaglandins are reported to either interfere with the progesterone secretion at the ovarian level (Hawk, 1967) or act as a luteolytic factor on the corpus luteum (Hubbard et al., 1978). In fact, luteolysis is implicated as the result of foreign body-provoked uterine inflammation (Ginther et al., 1966).

Increased vascularity and edema

Increased vascularity and alteration in membrane permeability of arterioles and venules reflect inflammatory reactions in the uterus caused by the IUD. Altered permeability leads to infiltration of inflammatory cells, which permeate the vessel walls and enter the endometrium (Kar, 1967). This permeability also affects the release of plasma exudates into the endometrial interstitium, thereby causing edema (Kar and Chandra, 1967).

Vascular changes in inflammatory reactions are governed by two types of mediators: (1) those that affect vasodilation, and (2) those that increase vascular permeability. The amount of plasma exudation is dependent on both types of mediators; the resulting edema can be modulated by either type (Williams and Peck, 1977).

Increase in mast cells—release of histamine and heparin

Prostaglandins, particularly of the E_1 and E_2 type, released as a result of IUD-induced inflammation, are reported to stimulate mast cells which, in turn, liberate histamine and heparin (Shaw, 1980). Since histamine has been implicated in increased vascular dilatation and permeability, its release may augment vascularity at the inflamed site. Heparin is known to impair blood coagulation, and this impairment may be responsible for increased blood flow locally. Mathur and Chowdhury (1968) have reported increased histamine content and the number of uterine mast cells in rats fitted with an IUD. However, in cows, no such effect on the mast cell count adjacent to the IUD-exposed endometrium has been observed (Hawk et al., 1968).

Activation of plasmin–plasminogen system—fibrinolysis

Extreme vascular permeability in IUD-exposed endometrium has been reported by Shaw et al. (1979). This appears to be a sign of persistent inflammatory reaction, caused by the IUD, and may lead to increased fibrinolytic activity in the endometrium (Liedholm and Astedt, 1976; Liedholm and Sjoberg, 1977; Shaw, 1980). Increased fibrinolytic potential of the IUD-exposed area reportedly results in the degradation of various coagulating factors (fibrinogen, prothrombin, labile factors, and antihemophilic globulins), consequently fibrin thrombosis does not occur (Shaw, 1980).

Fibrinolytic activity is believed to be regulated by two enzymes, plasmin and fibrinolysin, which are present in blood in the form of precursors, plasminogen and prefibrinolysin. The transformation of plasminogen into plasmin is brought about by activators (Casslen and Astedt, 1980; Shaw, 1980) and this activation process has been linked with an inflammatory reaction (Shaw, 1980).

Release of plasminogen activators and other enzymes

Plasminogen activators are reported to be released not only from the IUD-exposed autolyzing endometrium, but also from the inflammatory cells (Shaw et al., 1970). This may result in the generation of high plasmin activity at the IUD site.

Mehrotra and Srivastava (1982) have assessed (in vitro) the effect of rat uterine flushings of an IUD horn containing polymorphonuclear leukocytes on fibrin plates. The lysis of fibrin was enhanced significantly in plates exposed to uterine flushings from the IUD horn as compared to those from the non-IUD horn. This provides indirect evidence for the presence of a lytic enzyme, probably plasminogen activator, released by the breakdown of lysosomes present in leukocytes.

Parr and Shirley (1976) have demonstrated that leukocytes may also release certain other enzymes like β-galactosidase, the concentration of which, in the uterine fluid, reflects the extent of inflammation. This enzyme may be toxic to young embryos. However, the precise role of this enzyme in the action of an IUD is yet to be defined.

Role of anti-inflammatory and antifibrinolytic drugs

Use of anti-inflammatory drugs to check IUD-induced uterine inflammation was proposed by Parr and Segal (1966), who administered hydrocortisone to IUD-inserted rats. However, they failed to achieve the desired effect. Similarly, dexamethasone was found ineffective (Peppler and Molony, 1977). Aspirin and indomethacin, however, seemed to be better than corticoids (Chaudhuri, 1975; Williams and Peck, 1977). Indomethacin is reported to check inflammation by suppressing vasodilatory mediation, resulting in reduction of edema. (Williams and Peck, 1977). Our group (Srivastava and Mehrotra, 1978) induced partial inhibition of IUD-induced inflammatory changes in the rat uterus by administering two non-steroidal drugs, oxyphenbutazone and Curcumin (diferuloylmethane), and on this basis we support the hypothesis proposed by Parr (1969) that the genesis of IUD-induced inflammation is somewhat different from that caused by infective processes, or related to allergic reactions that can be checked by corticoids.

As stated earlier, the IUD induces local endometrial changes resulting in increased fibrinolytic activity (Casslen and Astedt, 1980). Interestingly, when the antifibrinolytic agent epsilonaminocaproic acid (EACA) was released through an IUD in the rabbit, the agent gave encouraging results in terms of counteracting the fibrinolytic activity and not influencing the contraceptive effect (Andrade et al., 1978).

Mehrotra and Srivastava (1982) have assessed three non-steroidal anti-inflammatory drugs: indomethacin, ibuprofen and naproxen-sodium on fibrin plates, pretreated with uterine flushings from luminal fluids of IUD horns. The enhanced lysis was partially checked by these drugs; the order of potentiality was indomethacin, ibuprofen, naproxen-sodium.

SUMMARY AND CONCLUSIONS

Insertion of an IUD is known to produce inflammatory reactions in the majority of animals, the intensity of which varies according to species. This reaction is indicated by the influx of polymorphs, macrophages, and other monocytes in the uterine endometrium and lumen. The influx of these inflammatory cells may be a consequence of a foreign body reaction, cell proliferation or transformation, increased vascularity and membrane permeability of the small capillaries, and/or the production/release of pro-inflammatory prostaglandins (PGI_2) into the uterine tissue. Other prostaglandins, particularly PGE_1 and PGE_2, stimulate the release of histamine and heparin from mast cells. Leukocytes and autolyzing endometrium release certain proteolytic enzymes such as plasminogen activator, which, in turn, activate the plasmin–plasminogen system and thus increase fibrinolytic activity in the uterine endometrium.

The use of non-steroidal anti-inflammatory drugs to ameliorate IUD-associated problems appears to be promising. Nevertheless, the combination of these drugs with antifibrinolytic agents may prove to have additional merits.

ACKNOWLEDGEMENTS

Authors are thankful to Drs V.P. Kamboj and Harish Chandra for critical evaluation and to Messrs P.K. Dasgupta, Arun, K. Srivastava and Ms Shakti Kichlu, for their help. Studies cited in this paper were supported by Ministry of Health and Family Welfare, Government of India.

References

Andrade, A.T.L., Shaw, S.T. Jr., Guerra, M.O. and Aaronson, D.E. (1978). Effect of epsilon-amino caproic acid on fertility in the rabbit. *J. Reprod. Fertil.*, **52**, 261-4

Bainton, D.F. (1980). The cells of inflammation; a general view In Glynn, L.E., Houck, and Weissmann, G. (eds). *The Cell Biology of Inflammation*. pp. 1-24. (Amsterdam Elsevier/ North Holland)

Casslen, B. and Astedt, B. (1980). IUDs and endometrial bleeding: biochemical aspects. In Hafez, E.S.E. and van Os, W.A.A. (eds.) *IUD Pathology and Management*, pp. 93-101. (Lancaster: MTP)

Chaudhuri, G. (1971). Intrauterine device: possible role of prostaglandin, a hypothesis. *Lancet*, **1**, 480

Chaudhuri, G. (1973). Release of prostaglandins by the IUCD. *Prostaglandins*, **3**, 773-84

Chaudhuri, G. (1975). Inhibition by aspirin and indomethacin of uterine hypertrophy induced by an IUD. *J. Reprod. Fertil.*, **43**, 77-81

Doyle, L.L. and Margolis, A.J. (1965). Intrauterine foreign body studies in rodents. In Segal, S.J., Southam, A.L. and Shafer, K.D. (eds.) *Proceedings of 2nd International Conference on Intrauterine Contraception*, pp. 185-197. (Amsterdam: Excerpta Medica)

Dumont, A.E. (1965). Fibroplasia: a sequel to lymphocyte exudation. In Zweifach, B.W., Grants, L. and McCluskey, R.T. (eds.) *The Inflammatory Process*, pp. 443-466. (New York City: Academic Press)

El Sahwi, S. and Moyer, D.L. (1971). The leukocytic response to an intrauterine foreign body in rabbit. *Fertil. Steril.*, **22**, 398-408

Gerrits, R.J., Hawk, H.W. and Stormshak, F. (1968). Fertility and corpus luteum characteristics in pigs with plastic devices in the uterine lumen. *J. Reprod. Fertil.*, **17**, 501-8

Ginther, O.J., Pope, A.L. and Casida, L.E. (1966). Local effect of an intrauterine plastic coil on the corpus luteum of the ewe. *J. Anim. Sci.*, **25**, 472-6

Greenwald, G.S. (1965). Interruption of pregnancy in the rat by a uterine suture. *J. Reprod. Fertil.*, **9**, 9-17

Hawk, H.W. (1967). Investigation into the antifertility effect of IUD in the ewe. *J. Reprod. Fertil.*, **14**, 49-59

Hawk, H.W., Conley, H.H. and Brinsfield, T.H. (1968). Studies on the antifertility effect of IUDs in cow. *Fertil. Steril.*, **19**, 411-18

Hubbard, C.J., Bo, W.J. and Krueger, W.A. (1978). The effect of the IUD and PGF_2^α on luteolysis in the pregnant hamster. *Biol. Reprod.*, **19**, 872-8

Janakiraman, K., Shukla, K.P., Gadgil, B.A. and Buch, N.C. (1970). Effect of intrauterine spirals and hormones on the uterine histology of the ovarectomized goat. *J. Reprod. Fertil.*, **11**, 145-8

Joshi, S.G. and Gunn, B.A. (1971). Effect of post-coital insertion of an intrauterine foreign body in rats. *Contraception*, **3**, 401-14

Kar, A.B. (1967). Mechanism of action of intrauterine contraceptive devices. In *Proceedings of 8th International Conference of IPPF*, Santiago, Chile. p. 393-402 (Hertford: Stephen Austin)

Kar, A.B. and Chandra, H. (1965). Uterine bleeding in rhesus monkeys after insertion of an intrauterine contraceptive device. *Indian J. Exp. Biol.*, **3**, 269-71

Kar, A.B. and Chandra, H. (1967). Uterine bleeding in prepubertal rhesus monkeys after intrauterine contraceptive device insertion. *Am. J. Obstet. Gynecol.*, **97**, 279-81

Lau, I.F., Saksena, S.K. and Chang, M.C. (1974). PGF in the uterine horns of mice with IUD. *J. Reprod. Fertil.*, **37**, 429-32

Ledger, W.J. and Bickley, J.E. (1966). Effect of plastic foreign body on the genital tract of the female rabbit. *Obstet. Gynecol. N.Y.*, **27**, 658–64

Liedholm, P. and Astedt, B. (1976). IUD increases the fibrinolytic activity of the rat endometrium at deciduation. *Experientia*, **32**, 226–7

Liedholm, P. and Sjoberg, N.O. (1977). Fibrinolytic activity in the rabbit uterus and its fluid with and without Cu-IUD. *Contraception*, **15**, 215–24

Martin, L. and Finn, C.A. (1979). Varying effects of an IUD on decidualization in mice. *J. Reprod. Fertil.*, **55**, 125–33

Mathur, V.S. and Chowdhury, R.R. (1968). The effect of an IUD (plastic) on the mast cell count in the rat uterus. *J. Reprod. Fertil.*, **15**, 135–8

Mehrotra, P.K. and Srivastava, K. (1982). Role of leucocytes, and plasminogen activators in IUDs mechanism of action: effect anti-inflammatory agents. *Contracept. Deliv. Syst.*, **2**, Abs. 180

Parr, E.L. (1969). The role of inflammation in the uterine weight caused by an IUD. *J. Reprod. Fertil.*, **18**, 221–6

Parr, E.L. (1970). Leucocytes and infertility. *J. Reprod. Fertil., Suppl.*, **10**, 153

Parr, E.L. and Segal, S.J. (1966). The effect of IUCD on the weight of the rat uterus. *Fertil. Steril.*, **17**, 648–53

Parr, E.L. and Shirley, R.L. (1976). Embryotoxicity of leukocyte extracts and its relationship to intrauterine contraception in humans. *Fertil. Steril.*, **27**, 1067–77

Peppler, R.D. and Molony, T. (1977). Effect of an anti-inflammatory compound on IUD effectiveness. *Anat. Rec.*, **187**, 775

Saksena, S.K., Lau, I.F. and Castracane, V.D. (1974). Prostaglandin mediated action of IUDs: 2F-prostaglandins (PGF) in the uterine horn of pregnant rats and hamsters with intrauterine devices. *Prostaglandins*, **5**, 97–106

Shaw, S.T. Jr. (1980). The enigma of uterine bleeding and IUDs. In Hafez, E.S.E. and van Os, W.A.A. (eds.) *IUD Pathology and Management.* p. 31.

Shaw, S.T. Jr., Cihak, R.W. and Moyer, D.L. (1970). Fibrin proteolysis in the monkey uterine cavity: variations with and without IUD. *Nature (London)*, **228**, 1097–8

Shaw, S.T. Jr., Macaulay, L.K. and Hohman, W.R. (1979). Morphology studies on IUD-induced metrorrhagia. II. Surface changes of endometrium and microscopic localization of bleeding sites. *Contraception*, **19**, 63–81

Srivastava, K. and Mehrotra, P.K. (1978). Effect of some nonsteroidal antiinflammatory agents on IUCD induced inflammation *Ind. J. Pharmacol.*, **10**, 21–25

Williams, J.J. and Peck, M.J. (1977). Role of PG-mediated vasodilation in inflammation. *Nature (London)*, **270**, 530–2

4
An intracervical device releasing norgestrel

M. ELSTEIN and I.D. NUTTALL

INTRODUCTION

The concept of the intracervical device (ICD) has been considered since the early 1970s, when it was reasoned that delivery of progestogens locally to the genital tract might overcome some of the problems associated with the oral intake of progestogens on a long-term basis.

The use of progestogen-only contraception was re-examined in the early 1960s, because of concern regarding the side-effects of the estrogen component of the combined pill (Rudel *et al.*, 1965). The evidence of thrombogenic effects of estrogen, in particular, resulted in an increasing acceptance of progestogens used alone especially for women at risk of these complications. In particular, the 19-norsteroid, norethisterone, and related steroids were used. This progestogen has a predominantly antiestrogenic action on the genital tract. Recently, there have been reports highlighting the association between an increased dose of progestogen and hypertension. The demonstrated reduction in high density lipoproteins may in turn be associated with an increased incidence of arterial disease (Kay, 1977; Larsson-Cohn, 1980). However, the effects of low dose progestogen-only contraception on these parameters is negligible. Additionally its effects on blood coagulation, carbohydrate metabolism and hepatic function are minimal compared to those of the combined formulations (Fotherby, 1976).

The problems concerning the oral delivery of progestogens, whose primary action was by inducing changes in the upper genital tract, were mainly concerned with a secondary effect on ovarian steroidogenesis. Variable suppression of ovulation, in up to 25% of cases, has been reported in several trials (Moghissi 1973; Elstein *et al.*, 1976). The inevitable consequence of this effect is a disruption of the normal menstrual pattern. The fluctuations in blood steroid levels, inevitable with intermittent dosing, may well be a major factor in producing this irregular pattern.

Any method of delivery of progestogens in which a fairly constant release of the drug is obtained might have several advantages. Firstly, a programmed release of the drug could be sustained over a long period.

Secondly, an optimal response, locally or systemically, could be obtained with a minimal quantity of drug which would reduce the problem of under- and over-dosing. Thirdly, there would be no need for daily intake of the drug which may be more convenient and acceptable.

Therefore, it appeared there was a need for the development of a low-dose progestogen delivery system which would provide a sustained and even release of the active drug into the cervical canal, thereby effecting a local sperm-blocking action. Since side-effects of steroid hormones are dose-dependent, a programmed low dose release would minimize their risk, provided the dose was within the range of effective contraceptive action.

Thus the development of the ICD stemmed from an awareness of these factors relating to the effectiveness and safety of the progestogens, and the concept that local delivery of these hormones provided a more rational method for their use than daily oral intake.

THE EFFECT OF PROGESTOGENS ON CERVICAL MUCUS

The composition of the cervical mucus visco-elastic gel is well documented (Elstein, 1978). The cervix has been described as a 'biological valve', which at certain stages of the menstrual cycle may facilitate or inhibit the free passage of spermatozoa (Moghissi, 1973). The alteration in composition of the mucus at various stages of the cycle has been assessed by investigations of its physical characteristics including volume, spinnbarkheit, viscosity and ferning.

Two clearly defined types of mucus are seen. Estrogenic (Type E) mucus has a low visco-elasticity. It has a high viscosity component, in which the glycoprotein mucin fibrils condense into micelles, and between these is the low viscosity cervical plasma (Odeblad, 1973). Just prior to ovulation, a further cascade of watery mucus is secreted (Type Es) which is optimally penetrable to sperm migration (Odeblad, 1978). It has been suggested that the penetration of mucus, produced by the cervix under estrogen dominance, is dependent simply upon the sperm's entry into this enclosed low viscosity component of the mucus. The action of pioneering spermatozoa may change the local environment of the mucus glycoprotein strands, facilitating the entry of other sperm (Katz et al., 1978). Following ovulation, progestogenic (Type G) mucus is secreted in response to corpus luteum dominance. This mucus has a smaller volume, due to reduction of its water content, and has a high visco-elasticity. The mucin fibrils in the micelles separate to form a densely entangled network which is impenetrable to sperm.

The relative amount of each type of mucus secreted is under the control of the hormone changes normally occurring in the menstrual cycle. Estrogen secretion in the preovulatory phase of the cycle is responsible for the production of a high percentage of Type E and the associated Type Es mucus, whilst the surge of progestogen normally apparent in the secretory phase stimulates a relative predominance of Type G mucus.

It follows that only in the preovulatory phase of the cycle is sperm penetration, resulting in fertilization, likely to occur. At other times the mucus, in the normal cycle, acts as a relative barrier to sperm penetration.

The action of exogenous progestogens on the cervical mucus has been well documented. It seemed logical that if mucus became impenetrable to sperm under the influence of endogenous progestogen production, then the intake of a daily dose of progestogens throughout the cycle might convert the mucus to a Type G (gestagenic) state. Rudel et al. (1965) and Martinez-Manautou et al. (1966) demonstrated that effective contraception was possible by using continuous chlormadinone acetate 0.5 mg daily, as a progestogen alone without inhibiting ovulation substantially. A contraceptive use effectiveness rate of 2.1 per 100 women-years was demonstrated. Ovulation was not inhibited to a significant degree and local genital tract changes were implicated. These were mainly in the form of the cervical mucus changes documented previously, the endometrium remaining secretory with a biphasic basal temperature chart and normal pregnanediol levels in the luteal phase.

Other studies using continuous low dose norethisterone and levonorgestrel as well as chlormadinone acetate demonstrated similar effects, although subtle changes in the endometrium and hypothalamic–pituitary function were noted (Zanartu et al., 1968; Foss et al., 1968; Howard et al., 1969). Kesseru et al. (1975) demonstrated that progesterone, levonorgestrel and cyproterone acetate had an in vitro effect on the physical properties of cervical mucus and sperm penetration. Progesterone was found to be the most active progestogen, but levonorgestrel also had a clear local effect. Cyproterone acetate did not demonstrate such action on the cervical mucus. The conclusion was that sperm migration was suppressed by a direct action of the steroid on the cervical mucus, which became opaque and thickened with a reduction in spinnbarkheit and crystallization.

Progestogens were thus shown to have a defined effect on cervical mucus as a result of their systemic action as well as by local diffusion. A subtle effect on hypothalamic-pituitary function occurred with oral low dose progestogens, as part of their mode of action, which might lead to this troublesome menstrual irregularity. which is a feature of many of the studies.

POSSIBLE BENEFITS OF AN ICD

A method of delivery of these low dose progestogens locally by a sustained programmed release mechanism, thereby minimizing alterations in hypothalamic–pituitary function, was therefore recognized as being highly desirable. Several methods of the local delivery of progestogens have been studied including vaginal rings (WHO, 1979), medicated intrauterine devices (Scommegna et al., 1970) and intracervical devices. Burton et al. (1980) summarized the positive assumptions that are made regarding the contraceptive effect of these locally delivered progestogens. Firstly, adequate progestogens should be released to cause a local effect on the reproductive tract, thereby providing the contraceptive action. Secondly, the systemic absorption of these progestogens should be minimal, in order to avoid disturbing pituitary-ovarian function. Thirdly, the locally released progestogens should inhibit sperm motility by changes in the cervical mucus. Consequently, low dose progestogens delivered directly to the cervix by a device seemed to satisfy these requirements.

The theoretical advantages of the ICDs over intrauterine devices might be a smaller menstrual loss with a lower incidence of pelvic inflammatory disease, as the device is not placed in the uterine cavity. Also, the device does not act as a potential abortifacient thereby increasing its acceptability to certain religious groups. Finally, the device could be inserted by para-medical workers with a smaller incidence of uterine perforation and mis-placement than an intrauterine device.

It therefore seemed that with these advantages in mind, as well as the theoretical benefits of local delivery of a low dose progestogen, development of the intracervical device would produce a valuable alternative contraceptive method.

DEVELOPMENT OF THE ICD—ANIMAL STUDIES

Initial animal studies (Glass and Morris, 1972; Greenhill and Glass, 1972) demonstrated the effect of chlormadinone acetate impregnated silicone rubber devices in the New Zealand white rabbit cervix. The device, containing 15% chlormadinone by weight and being 0.9 cm in length, was sutured into the cervix of one uterine horn at laparotomy. There was a clear inhibitory effect on sperm transport in the horn under study compared with its contralateral control. A follow-up long-term study over 6 months using the same technique, and removing the devices every 2 months, showed some degenerative changes in the endocervical tissue, but no inflammatory reaction.

Other studies examined the release rates of norethisterone and levonorgestrel from ICDs in similar rabbits, together with the local and systemic drug-related changes. Differing release rates of the drugs were obtained. The reproductive tracts in most rabbits were normal apart from a mild granulation reaction related to the suture used to hold the device in place. There were no obvious treatment-related changes. Focal hyperplasia of the uterine mucosa was noted, but these were also seen when oral progestogens were administered. Estimation of drug release rates suggested satisfactory levels in the high dose models, compared with the target in the human of release rates of 25 μg per day of levonorgestrel and 50 μg per day of norethisterone, respectively (Moghissi et al., 1977).

Trials were also performed with Patas monkeys using a scaled down version of the human intracervical device (Burton et al., 1980). The devices were designed with high and low release rates of norgestrel. They were coated with a layer of pure silicone rubber to control the drug release rate and protect the cervical surface. After approximately 3 months the monkeys were killed. Histological examination of the endometrium of some of the monkeys in both groups of release rate levels showed stromal hyperplasia. The glandular epithelium was hyperplastic and in some cases there were mitotic figures lining the stroma. Examination of the cervix of some monkeys also showed hyperplastic changes with small amounts of squamous metaplasia occasionally seen. Radioimmunoassay estimation of progesterone levels suggested ovulation was generally occurring. During the trial the cervical mucus was examined at mid-cycle. The results suggested that levonorgestrel induced progestational changes in the cervical mucus.

These animal studies suggested that satisfactory release rates of progestogen from an ICD could be obtained using animal models, but there were some histological changes related to treatment which might cause concern. Questions were raised regarding the suitability of the monkey species used and the World Health Organisation (WHO) determined to find further animal species which would more clearly relate to the human model, where there is a straight endocervical canal (WHO, 1978). This feature of the animal studies will be further discussed in relation to the clinical trials.

DEVELOPMENT OF THE ICD—CLINICAL TRIALS

A number of clinical studies using the ICDs have been performed over the last decade, using different progestogens including progesterone, chlormadinone acetate and, more recently, levonorgestrel. This latter potent 19-norsteroid has been found to be the most suitable steroid for use in this type of device. Studies have also been performed using the spermicidal agents, quinine sulfate and emetine. Most recent studies have been performed by WHO in parallel with the National Institutes of Health, USA.

Cohen *et al.* (1970) formulated a device consisting of medical grade Silastic tubing 22 mm in length, holding 20–30 mg of progesterone at a release rate of 250 µg per 24 hours. The device had an outer diameter of 2.61 mm and was attached to a nylon thread for identification purposes. Each subject acted as her own control and was studied during pretreatment and treatment cycles. Six subjects during seven cycles showed convincing evidence of a change from estrogenic to gestagenic mucus, as determined by alterations in its physical properties as described above. Although not suitable for long-term use, these devices gave the impetus to research for a more sophisticated intracervical device.

Glass and Morris (1972) used cervical stem inserts releasing different rates of chlormadinone acetate over a period of 3 weeks. They showed a release rate of 150 µg chlormadinone acetate per day which was sufficient to change the cervical mucus into the progestational type without affecting systemic hormonal function. Lower release rates did not affect the mucus. The authors' conclusion was that the introduction of progestogens directly into the cervix was the most efficient way of preventing sperm migration thereby fulfilling the earlier criteria of Burton regarding the lowest dose of drug producing a contraceptive effect without causing systemic changes.

In 1972, WHO instituted a program to develop an ICD which could cause local genital tract action without suppression of ovulation. An inert device was developed and subjected to clinical trial. This device was 1.5 cm long and consisted of a small cylinder of polypropylene, and was split at the upper end to form two branches which lay in the transverse plane of

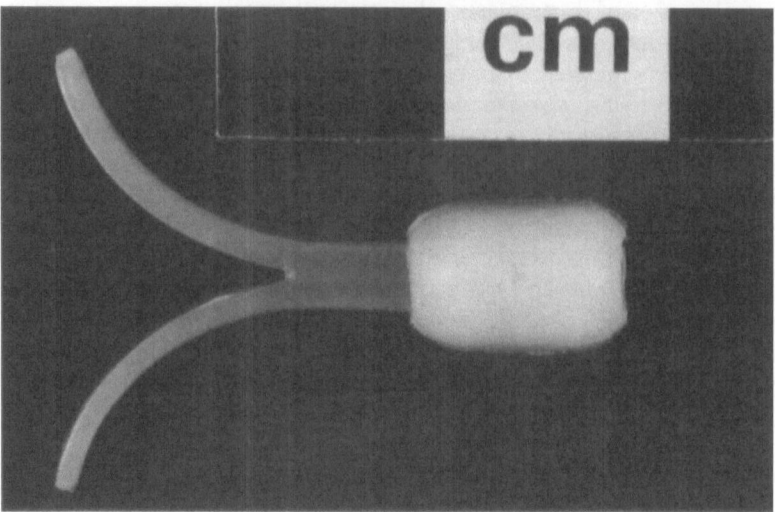

Figure 4.1 The WHO intracervical device showing the L-norgestrel impregnated polysilicone reservoir

the uterus at the level of the internal os. There was a polysilicone reservoir surrounding the lower stem which contained the active drug (Figure 4.1). This would allow a sustained release of the drug into the cervical mucus.

As stated earlier, clinical trials of primitive active devices used progesterone, chlormadinone acetate and norethisterone, but WHO initially concentrated on spermicidal-releasing devices using quinine sulfate. Trials with these devices releasing 20 μg per day of quinine sulfate demonstrated an inhibition of sperm migration in 80% of the postcoital tests, with no local or systemic adverse reactions. At the same time, the National Institutes of Health, USA, were developing a progestogen device which released levonorgestrel 20-25 μg per day over a prolonged period. Initial *in vitro* studies suggested that further development of the device was worthwhile (Moghissi *et al.*, 1977).

In the early WHO trials there was a high expulsion rate (27.8%) of the inert device, especially in nulliparous women (Buckingham *et al.*, 1977). A modified device (prototype II) was developed, in which the arms were stiffer and 2 mm longer than in the original model. A statistically improved retention rate was obtained with the modified device, and showed it to be suitable for further development.

At this stage, the previously mentioned Patas monkey trials were reported, noting endocervical metaplasia in some cases. The WHO Task Force considered that these changes might have occurred because the device abutted directly onto the surface epithelium of the cervical canal. Initially, a search was made for an animal model in which the cervical canal more closely resembled the human, so that further studies could be performed. It was felt that the problem would probably not occur in the human because the device was not in direct contact with the cervical epithelium.

As no satisfactory or practical animal model could be found, although the baboon was considered, it was decided to investigate women who were undergoing hysterectomy for other reasons. The broad aims of the study were to ascertain whether the ICD has an adverse effect on the histology and bacteriology of the cervical canal, as well as studying the effect of levonorgestrel-releasing devices on sperm migration (WHO, 1978). The study was deemed crucial for further development of intracervical devices in view of these animal toxicological findings, and the feasibility of this approach to the control of fertility needed to be established.

HYSTERECTOMY STUDY

This study had two major objectives. Firstly, whether the intracervical device had an adverse effect on the histology and bacteriology of the cervical canal and uterine cavity; and secondly, whether the release of norgestrel 20-25 μg per day would affect the cervical mucus characteristics sufficiently to inhibit sperm migration through the cervical canal. This report relates to a study performed in Manchester, England.

Women aged between 20 and 40 years, who were listed to undergo routine hysterectomy, were recruited. Pathological lesions affecting the cervical canal and lower portion of the uterine cavity were excluded. Subjects recruited had previously been sterilized or were using a barrier method of contraception. They had regular 28-day menstrual cycles and showed ovulatory cervical mucus in the control phase. The patients were allocated into three groups. One group had a levonorgestrel-releasing device fitted after a control cycle. The second group had an inert device and there was a control group who had no device placed.

During the control cycle, the cervical mucus was assessed on alternate days in the periovulatory phase. Physical characteristics of volume, clarity, spinnbarkheit, viscosity and ferning were determined. At the same time, postcoital tests were performed and, where appropriate, sperm penetration was assessed using the Kremer capillary technique.

The ICD was fitted after the first cycle and subjects were investigated in the manner described above for the following two cycles.

After hysterectomy, the uterus was immediately opened under sterile conditions and punch biopsies were taken along the endocervical canal and uterine cavity as described by Sparks et al. (1977). Cultures of these samples were made under aerobic and anaerobic conditions using the same procedures. The uterus was fixed and a detailed histological study of the endocervical canal in particular was performed.

The results of this study indicated that the active progestogen-releasing ICD converted ovulatory mucus to the gestational type in 80% of cases, which inhibited sperm mobility and survival as determined by the postcoital test (Tables 4.1, 4.2). There was no such conversion noted in control patients or those using the inert device. These changes certainly gave enough evidence to warrant further assessment of the ICD as a fertility–regulating agent.

However, bacteriological and histological assessment of the uterus after

Table 4.1 Cervical score measured by the Insler method (Insler, V., Melmud, H., Eichenbrenner, I., Serr, D. and Lunenfeld, B. (1972). The cervical score. *Int. J. Gynaec. Obstet.*, **10**, 223)

	Inert device		Active device	
	Control cycle	Test cycle	Control cycle	Test cycle
Range	4-12	0-10	7-11	0-5
n	10	16	10	17
Mean	8.6	5.0	10.0	1.0

Table 4.2 Postcoital test score (WHO Task Force method)

	Inert device		Active device	
	Control cycle	Test cycle	Control cycle	Test cycle
Range	3-7	0-6	2-9	0-5
n	8	12	9	14
Mean	5.0	2.3	5.9	0.4

hysterectomy did give some cause for concern. In many of the specimens where an ICD had been present, there was clear evidence of reserve cell hyperplasia and focal metaplasia and some focal inflammatory changes (Table 4.3). The significance of these changes is not clear, as similar changes are seen when an intrauterine device has been fitted, although usually over a longer time-scale (Buckley, personal communication). It is also not clear whether these changes occur in the normal uterus, as such intensive histology is not usually performed. Also, in a limited study of 3 months, extrapolation to longer-term use of the device is not possible. A more diffuse metaplasia which might occur could lead to relative infertility and susceptibility to infection.

The bacteriological study (Table 4.4) suggested that the cervical barrier was broken by the intracervical device and bacteriological colonization of the uterine cavity occurred in approximately 60% of cases with the device *in situ*. Organisms ranged from commensals such as *Lactobacilli*, to pathogenic bacteria such as *Staphylococcus aureus* and *Bacteroides*. The uterine cavity is normally a sterile environment (Sparks *et al.*, 1977) and coloniza-

Table 4.3 Number of patients in each group with histological changes

Active device	Sup. ulceration	2
	Mild inflammatory changes	4
	CIN II	1
	CIN I	1
Inert device	Sup. ulceration	1
	Mild inflammatory changes	4
	CIN I	1
Control	Mild inflammatory changes	3
	CIN III	1

Table 4.4 Number of patients in each group showing bacteriological colonization of the lower and upper genital tract

Site		Active	Inert	Control
H V S	Growth	6	5	3
	No growth	3	4	5
Cervix	Growth	6	6	4
	No growth	3	3	4
Uterus	Heavy growth	2	4	0
	Light growth	3	2	2
	No growth	4	3	6

tion to this degree suggests that even though the ICD is not placed in the uterine cavity, any device which bridges the cervical barrier allows passage of bacteria into the uterine cavity which would not normally be present.

The broad conclusions from this study were that, although the progestogen-releasing ICD appeared to act effectively in inhibiting sperm migration through the cervix, the local side-effects might be too great to allow its development to continue. A device which facilitates bacteriological colonization of the uterine cavity might activate local tissue responses. In the long-term this could lead to clinical disease, and would not offer the advantages initially perceived.

CONCLUSIONS

The ICD was developed in response to a concern regarding the problems related to delivery of progestogens orally, with all the pharmacodynamic and clinical problems that might result. A non-coitally related device delivering a sustained low dose release of progestogen directly to the genital tract seemed to offer certain advantages over conventional dosing.

Although the delivery of progestogens locally by the ICD might be a realistic proposition in the inhibition of sperm migration, local effects of the device on the cervical canal would mitigate against its long-term development and pessimism has been expressed regarding the long-term future of this device (WHO, 1979).

It may be that the local delivery of progestogens to the genital tract may be better served by devices such as the medicated vaginal ring, which seems to hold more promise and these are being developed further.

ACKNOWLEDGEMENTS

The study described was supported by the World Health Organisation,

Special Programme of Research, Development and Research Training in Human Reproduction, Project No. 78034.
Dr I.D. Nuttall was the recipient of a Research Fellowship from Schering Pharmaceutical Limited, Sussex, England, during part of these studies.

References

Buckingham, M.S., Everitt, J. and Elstein, M. (1977). An inert intracervical contraceptive device—a preliminary clinical trial. In Insler, V. and Bettendorf, G. (eds.) *The Uterine Cervix in Reproduction.* p. 277. (Stuttgart: George Thieme)

Burton, F.G., Skiens, W.E., Duncan, G.W. and Sikar, M.R. (1980). Medicated intracervical devices. In Hafez, E.S.E. and van Os, W.A.A. (eds.) *Biodegradeables and Delivery Systems for Contraception.* p. 139. (Lancaster: MTP Press)

Cohen, M.R., Pandya, G.N. and Scommegna, A. (1970). The effects of an intracervical steroid releasing device on the cervical mucus. *Fertil. Steril.*, **21**, 715-23

Elstein, M. (1978). Functions and physical properties of mucus in the female genital tract. *Br. Med. Bull.*, **34**, 83-8

Elstein, M., Briston, P.G., Hewitt, K.J., Kirk, D. and Miller, H. (1976). The effect of daily norethisterone (0.35 mg) on cervical mucus and on urinary LH, pregnanediol and oestrogen levels. *Br. J. Obstet. Gynaecol.*, **83**, 165-8

Foss, G.L., Svendsen, E.K., Fotherby, K. and Richards, D.J. (1968). Contraceptive action of continuous low doses of norgestrel. *Br. Med. J.*, **4**, 489-91

Fotherby, K. (1976). Low doses of gestagens as fertility regulating agents. In Dieczfalusy, E. (ed.) *Regulation of Human Fertility.* p. 283. (Copenhagen: Scriptor)

Glass, R.H. and Morris, J.M. (1972). Antifertility effects of an intracervical progestational device. *Biol. Reprod.*, **7**, 160-5

Greenhill, A. and Glass, R.H. (1972). Histologic effects of intracervical chlormadinone impregnated silastic devices in rabbits. *Contraception*, **6**, 287-94

Howard, G., Elstein, M., Blair, M. and Morris, N.F. (1969). Low dose continuous chlormadinone acetate as an oral contraceptive. *Lancet*, **2**, 24-6

Katz, D.F., Mills, R.N., and Pritchett, T.R. (1978). The movement of human spermatozoa in cervical mucus. *J. Reprod. Fertil.*, **53**, 258-65

Kay, C.R. (1977). Effect on hypertension and benign breast disease of progestogen component in combined oral contraceptives. Royal College of General Practitioners Oral Contraceptive Study. *Lancet*, **1**, 624

Kesseru, E., Camacho-Ortega, P., Laudahn, G. and Schopflin, G. (1975). *In vitro* action of progestogens on sperm migration in human cervical mucus. *Fertil. Steril.*, **26**, 57-61

Larsson-Cohn, U. (1980). Effects of some ethinyl oestradiol/norgestrel combinations on lipid metabolism. In Newton, J.R., Jacob, H.S. and Caldwell, A.D.S. (eds.) *Workshop on Fertility Control, Royal Society of Medicine (International Congress and Symposium)*, No. 31, p. 57. (London: Academic Press)

Martinez-Manautou, J., Cortez, V., Giner, J., Aznar, R., Casasola, J. and Rudel, H.W. (1966). Low doses of progestogen as an approach to fertility control. *Fertil. Steril.*, **17**, 49-57

Moghissi, K.S. (1973). Sperm migration through the human cervix. In Elstein, M., Moghissi, K.S. and Borth, R. (eds.) *Cervical Mucus in Human Reproduction.* p. 128. (Copenhagen: Scriptor)

Moghissi, K.S., Burton, F.G., Skiens, W.E., Leininger, R.I., Sikov, M.R., Duncan, G.W. and Smith, L.G. (1977). An intracervical contraceptive device. In Gabelnick, H.L. (ed.) *Drug Delivery Systems.* p. 79. (Washington DC: US Department of Health, Education and Welfare, Government Printing Office)

Odeblad, E. (1973). Biophysical techniques of assessing cervical mucus and microstructure of cervical epithelium. In Elstein, M., Moghissi, K.S. and Borth, R. (eds.) *Cervical Mucus in Human Reproduction.* p. 58. (Copenhagen: Scriptor)

Odeblad, E. (1978). Cervical factor. *Contr. Gynecol. Obstet.*, **4**, 132-42

Rudel, H.W., Martinez-Manautou, J. and Maqueo-Topete, M. (1965). The role of progestogens in the hormonal control of fertility. *Fertil. Steril.*, **16**, 158.

Scommegna, A., Pandya, G.N., Christ, M., Lee, A.W. and Cohen, M.R. (1970). Intrauterine administration of progesterone by a slow releasing device. *Fertil. Steril.*, **21,** 201-10

Sparks, R.A., Purrier, B.G.A., Watt, P.J. and Elstein, M. (1977). The bacteriology of the cervix and uterus. *Br. J. Obstet. Gynaecol.*, **84,** 701-4

WHO Special Programme of Research, Development and Research Training in Human Reproduction. Seventh Annual Report (1978). *Intracervical Devices.* (Geneva: WHO)

WHO Special Programme of Research, Development and Research Training in Human Reproduction. Eighth Annual Report (1979). *Intracervical Devices.* p. 76. (Geneva: WHO)

Zanartu, J., Rodriquez-Moore, G., Pupkin, M., Salas, O., Guerrero, R. (1968). Antifertility effect of continuous low-dosage oral progestogen therapy. *Br. Med. J.*, **2,** 263-6

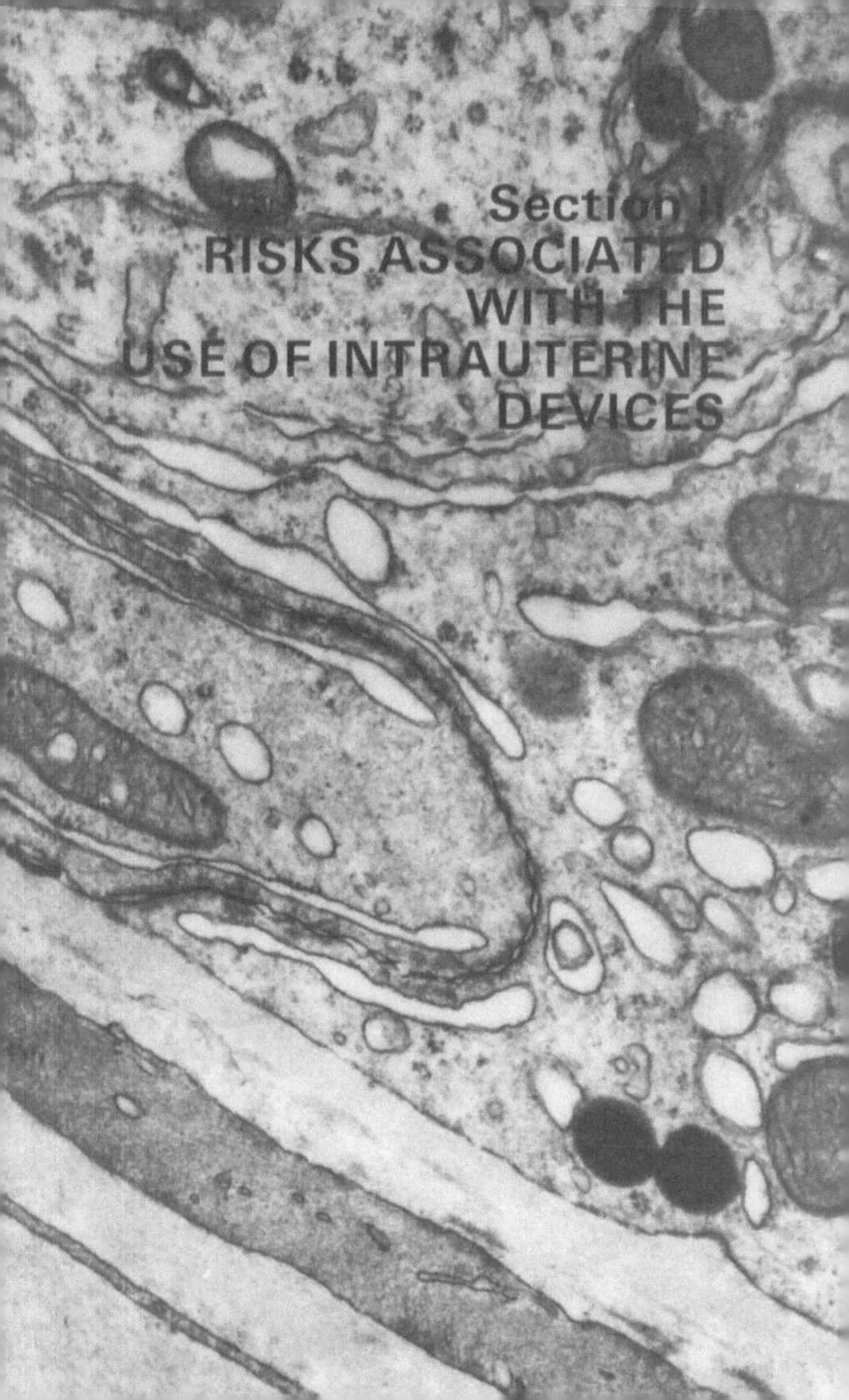

Section II
RISKS ASSOCIATED
WITH THE
USE OF INTRAUTERINE
DEVICES

5
Risk factors for pelvic inflammatory disease in IUD users

M. KOŽUH-NOVAK, L. ANDOLŠEK, H. HREN-VENCELJ, M. GUBINA
and B. KRALJ

Pelvic inflammatory disease is an infrequent side-effect of intrauterine device use. The cumulative discontinuation rate for PID in comparative trials ranges from 2 per 100 users, during the first year after insertion (Luukkainen et al., 1979) to 0.1 per 100 users after 2 years of IUD use (WHO, 1982), depending on the research group, the criteria for PID diagnosis, and the type of IUD.

An increasing number of studies in the past decade have been undertaken to determine the prevalence of PID in IUD users, the potential severity of the disease, and its health and economic consequences.

In several studies, PID was found to be 2.0–7.9 times more frequent in IUD users than in controls. Of the methodological difficulties in investigating this problem, the most serious is the accuracy of clinical diagnosis, also several confounding variables are rarely included, and formation of an appropriate control group is difficult.

In a review article, Senanayake and Kramer (1980) suggested that after oral contraceptive users had been excluded from the control group, the risk for PID in IUD users was smaller (1.6–4.0) than previous comparisons had demonstrated. In spite of this finding, PID remains a major concern in IUD use.

As IUD users tend to continue wearing IUDs until the menopause and are therefore at long-term risk for developing PID, two questions arise:

(1)   What factors contribute to the development of PID in IUD users.
(2)   Do certain events during IUD use predict severe episodes of PID?

Several studies demonstrate that women at risk for developing PID are less than 30 years of age, with several sexual partners, and of low socioeconomic status (Eschenbach, 1980; Faulkner and Ory, 1976; Weström et al., 1976; Wright and Laemmle, 1968). Additional factors may contribute to the development of PID in IUD users.

Potential risk factors for PID in IUD users are of three types: (1) user-related; (2) IUD-related; and (3) etiological agent-related. This schematic classification is an artificial one, however, as PID is likely to have multiple causes (Holmes et al., 1980).

USER-RELATED RISK FACTORS

Sociodemographic aspects

Are women who select an IUD different from others?

According to Edelman *et al.* (1982), investigators of PID have neglected the findings of authors, demonstrating that differences exist among women selecting different contraceptive methods. Consequently, it is possible that women who select an IUD already carry a certain risk factor when the device is inserted. Burkman (1981) tested the hypothesis that women who had suffered from PID were less likely to select an IUD. He separately analyzed a group of women with a history of PID and a group of women without PID. He found a higher relative risk (RR) for PID in IUD users who had suffered from PID previously (2.1) than in those women in whom the first PID episode was observed during IUD use (1.2).

A similar finding is reported by the same author in women who had more than one sexual partner. RR for PID in IUD users with more than one partner was 2.6, while in those with one partner only, the relative risk was 1.7. The author explains the difference by a greater tendency of women with more partners to develop PID, regardless of other factors.

A lower prevalence of PID in oral contraceptive users found in some studies suggested to Holmes *et al.* (1980) that oral contraceptives could be administered to women recovering from the first PID episode to prevent its recurrence.

Are IUD users sexually more active than OC users?

Adams *et al.* (1978) found that women using oral contraceptives did not show a rise in female-initiated sexual activity at mid-cycle. The micelle arrangement of the mucin allows sperm penetration in mid-cycle but not at other times (Odevald, 1976); similar restraints may apply to bacteria (Sparks *et al.*, 1981). The ability of several species of pathogenic bacteria to migrate through mid-cycle mucus adhering to IUD tails has been shown (Parrier *et al.*, 1979).

If oral contraceptive users have sexual intercourse in the mid-cycle period less frequently than do IUD users, it is possible that this factor also contributes to the difference in prevalence of PID.

Age and parity

The highest PID rates have been found among sexually active women between ages 15 and 25 (Eschenbach, 1980).

Are these findings valid for IUD users as well?

IUD users do not differ from the total population as regards the distribution of PID rates by age-groups (Burkman, 1981; Faulkner and Ory, 1976; Kaufman *et al.*, 1980). We have tried to answer the question in a case-control study comparing the characteristics of IUD users who had developed PID requiring IUD removal with the characteristics of other IUD users (Kozuh-Novak and Andolsek, 1982). For this purpose, the IUD records of the Family Planning Institute and the clinical records of the Department of Obstetrics and Gynecology in Ljubljana were used. The data were collected from the records of 8088 women who had the first IUD insertion between 1964 and 1972. Thus, IUDs were in the uterus from 1 to 16 years. The follow-up rate was approximately 98% for the first year.

After 8 years, the follow-up rate was still 80%, and the continuation rate was 50%. During the observation period, IUDs were removed from 378 women because of PID. Nine gynecologists participated in the study. The diagnosis of PID (endometritis, adnexitis with or without abscess formation, and pelvic peritonitis) was based mainly on physical examination and laboratory findings. We classified as PID any episode requiring antibiotic treatment for a painful and/or enlarged uterus or adnexa. To determine characteristics among women in whom the IUD was removed for PID and other IUD users, each woman with PID was matched with a control selected among the 8088 IUD users. The controls were women in whom an IUD had been inserted at the same time as an IUD was inserted in a woman who subsequently developed PID and who had the IUD *in situ* for the same length of time. This method of comparison yielded 378 women with PID and 381 controls.

Among the PID cases, there were 57 women who needed surgical treatment because of a severe PID. All were hospitalized for 6-99 days; the mean hospital stay was 25.6 days. The women were grouped according to whether they had severe or mild PID; 14 women were excluded because it was not clear to which group they belonged. The age distribution of the three groups of women is presented in Table 5.1.

The women with mild PID were slightly younger than the controls at the time of IUD insertion, but the difference was not significant. Women with severe PID were significantly ($p < 0.01$) younger at the insertion of the IUD than those in the control group. The women do not differ significantly in education, number of children, number of induced abortions, use of contraceptives before IUD insertion, type of device used, and preinsertion PID episodes.

Parity appeared to be less important than was thought earlier (Senanayake and Kramer, 1980).

IUD-RELATED RISK FACTORS

Duration of IUD use and severity of disease

Vessey *et al.* followed 17 032 women for at least 6 years (1981). They found that PID rates diminished during the observation period. Burkman (1981) looked at the time of IUD insertion, the total duration of IUD use, and the occurrrence of PID severe enough to require hospitalization. Using a long-linear model he did not find a correlation between the duration of IUD use and the prevalence of PID. The duration of IUD use was not

Table 5.1 Comparison by age and insertion of women from whom the IUD was removed for PID and controls

Age	PID		Controls
(years)	mild	severe	
≤ 19	5	0	11
20–24	65	17	79
25–29	95	24	96
30–34	92	9	106
35–39	40	7	72
≥ 40	10	0	17
Total	307	57	381

described. Kaufman *et al.* (1980) found the risk for PID in women with an IUD *in situ* for more than 5 years to be 12.9 and in those with an IUD *in situ* for less than 5 years, 5.7. It should be mentioned, however, that their sample was small and the diagnostic criteria were not clearly defined.

Phaosavaski *et al.* (1975) evaluated tubal changes in 200 women undergoing sterilization. 101 of these women had used IUDs for varying periods of time. The authors analyzed tubal changes in relation to duration of IUD use and concluded that the tubal changes increase with duration of IUD use.

We compared the duration of IUD use to the severity of PID (Kozuh-Novak and Andolsek, 1982) (Table 5.2). A significantly larger number of IUD users with severe PID had had the IUD *in situ* for more than 5 years as compared to women with mild PID (RR = 1.8). Similar results were seen in a survey of women having IUD-related complications requiring hospitalization (Danev and Kozuh-Novak, 1983). Data were collected from 15 hospitals in Slovenia. In 1981 152 users were hospitalized for PID. Duration of hospital treatment was the criterion used to determine the severity of PID. Table 5.3 shows the distribution of IUD users by duration of use and by duration of hospital treatment. Fourteen women (9.2%) for whom the data were incomplete were excluded from analysis. Of the remaining 139 women, those with an IUD *in situ* for more than 5 years were hospitalized for a significantly longer period of time. RR for severe PID in women with a long-term IUD use (more than 5 years) is 3.9, in comparison with women using an IUD for a shorter time. It should be noted, however, that the

Table 5.2 Duration of use in women having an IUD removed for PID

Years of use	Mild PID	%	Severe PID	%
≤ 1	76	24.7	9	15.8
2–5	139	45.3	23	40.4
6–9	68	22.1	19	33.3
10–12	24	7.8	6	10.5
Total	307	100	57	100

Table 5.3 Duration of hospital treatment for PID and duration of IUD use in 139 IUD users

IUD use (years)	Hospital treatment (days)				
	1-14	%	15+	%	Total
<5	70	83.3	31	56.4	101
>5	14	16.7	24	43.6	38
Total	84	100	55	100	139

$\chi^2 = 12.3; p < 0.001; RR = 3.9$

diagnosis of PID is not uniform in all hospitals and that it is generally based on clinical and laboratory procedures.

Maqueo *et al.* (1979) performed histologic examinations of Fallopian tube tissue obtained during sterilization procedures in 225 women. RR for acute changes in IUD users was 1.5. When comparing the severity of disease, he found marked inflammation in 25% of IUD users and in only 4.5% of non-users. According to Senanayake and Kramer (1980), the validity of these findings is limited because the definition of PID was not specified.

The hypothesis that PID tends to be more severe in IUD users is also supported by studies in which an elevated body temperature was a key criterion for PID diagnosis. Wright and Laemmle (1968) reported attack rates per 100 women-years of 6.6 for IUD users and 1.3 for oral contraceptive users. Targum and Wright (1974) reported that the RR for IUD users was 9.3, Faulkner and Ory (1976) found that the RR was 5.1 in febrile IUD users and 2.7 in afebrile users.

Events during IUD use

Theorizing that a careful follow-up of the IUD users might allow intervention before the onset of severe PID, we considered whether women who

Table 5.4 Bleeding episodes during IUD use and severity of PID in women whose IUD was removed for PID, and controls

Bleeding episodes	PID				Controls
	Mild	RR	Severe	RR	
0	129		28		205
1-2	121	1.5	23	1.3	128
3+	57	1.9	6	0.9	48
Total	307*		57†		381

*$\chi^2 = 10.39$	†$\chi^2 = 1.4$
2 d.f.	2 d.f.
$p < 0.01$	NS

Table 5.5 Intermenstrual spotting episodes during IUD use and severity of PID in women whose IUD was removed for PID, and controls

Spotting episodes	PID				Controls
	Mild	RR	Severe	RR	
0	67		12		118
1–2	82	2.6	18	1.6	108
3+	158	1.8	27	1.7	155
Total	307*		57†		381

* $\chi^2 = 11.3$
2 d.f.
$p < 0.001$

† $\chi^2 = 2.31$
2 d.f.
N.S.

had an IUD removed for PID had experienced more bleeding, spotting, and PID episodes during IUD use than had other IUD users (Kozuh-Novak and Andolsek, 1982).

A significant difference in the incidence of bleeding episodes was found between women with mild PID and controls (Table 5.4). However, no significant differences were seen in bleeding episodes in the women with severe PID and controls. Analysis of spotting episodes (Table 5.5) revealed a significant difference between women with mild PID and controls.

Comparing PID episodes during IUD use in women with PID and controls, a significant difference was found (Table 5.6).

Since frequent follow-up visits might exert an influence on the recording of bleeding, spotting, and PID episodes during IUD use, we looked at how many women with severe PID and how many with mild PID came for a gynecological check-up at least once a year. In the women with mild PID, 57% came regularly, and in the women with severe PID, 46% came regularly. The difference is not significant.

Table 5.6 PID episodes before IUD removal in women whose IUD was removed for PID, and controls

PID episodes	PID				Controls
	Mild	RR	Severe	RR	
0	28		8		296
1–2	250	33.0	48	22.2	80
3+	29	61.3	1	7.4	5
Total	307*		57†		381

* $\chi^2 = 322.1$
2 d.f.
$p < 0.001$

† $\chi^2 = 96.9$
2 d.f.
$p < 0.001$

Table 5.7 Type of IUD and severity of PID in women whose IUD was removed for PID, and controls

IUD	PID				Controls	
	Mild	%	Severe	%	n	%
LLD	136	44.3	15	26.3	169	44.4
LLC	57	18.6	9	15.8	68	17.8
M-DEV	58	18.9	6	10.5	66	17.3
Margulies	39	12.7	18	31.6	22	5.7
Others	17	5.5	9	15.8	56	14.6
Total	307	100	57*	100	381	100

* $\chi^2 = 41.4$
4 d.f.
$p < 0.001$

Type of IUD

In prospective studies (Edelman *et al.*, 1982; Vessey *et al.*, 1981) in which PID rates for various types of IUD were followed up for 6–8 years, no significant differences were found. Kaufman *et al.* (1980) found a borderline significant difference between the Cu 7 and three other types of IUD, but their findings are unconvincing, because of the high percentage of unknown types of IUD involved in their study. Burkman *et al.* (1981), comparing PID rates for Lippes D and Cu 7, found no significant differences between the two IUDs. In our study (Kozuh-Novak and Andolsek, 1982) no significant differences among various types of IUDs were found when we compared mild PID cases with controls. However, we noticed that the Margulies spiral was the device most frequently associated with severe PID (Table 5.7). The RR for this device in severe PID was 9.2 compared to controls and 4.2 compared to Lippes Loop D.

Is reinsertion of the IUD connected with an increased risk?

Burkman (1981) found that the RR for developing PID in the first 30 days post-IUD insertion was 3.8 times greater than in subsequent periods. Similar findings are also reported by Nilsson *et al.* (1981), who analyzed prevalence of bacteria on IUDs removed for PID. Burkman (1981) also found that the increased risk for PID persists for 12 months after discontinuation of IUD use. Further studies in this field will have to take into account three factors.

(1) The reason for removing the previous IUD. In a woman who has changed her IUD because of a side-effect (bleeding, pregnancy, expulsion), more problems may be expected with the next IUD than in a woman whose previous IUD was removed for other reasons.

(2) The interval between removal of an IUD and insertion of another. Since studies show that copper IUDs are effective much longer than was expected at first (Kozuh-Novak and Andolsek, 1980; Lippes, 1975;

71

Zipper *et al.*, 1976), the question arises whether the risk with a periodical change of the IUD (entailing a risk for PID or accidental pregnancy) would be greater than that of long-term uninterrupted use.

(3) On the other hand, if long-term users are, as our study suggested, at a higher risk for PID (Kozuh-Novak and Andolsek, 1982), duration of previous IUD use as well as the number of PID episodes before reinsertion will have to be taken into account (Westrom *et al.*, 1976).

AGENT-RELATED RISK FACTORS

PID has a polymicrobial etiology. Changes in the genital tract with an IUD, and a higher incidence of PID in IUD users has led investigators to search for a possible difference in the prevalence of micro-organisms in these women as compared to others.

Watt *et al.* (1981) analyzed bacterial flora in the cervix and fornix of 1498 young women. In 46% an abnormal vaginal discharge was found. A significantly greater quantity of anaerobic bacteroides species was found in IUD users compared to non-users. Goldacre *et al.* (1979) isolated anaerobes more frequently from the vaginas of IUD users than from non-IUD users. Holmes *et al.* (1980) suggested that non-specific vaginitis is significantly more frequent in IUD users.

Sparks *et al.* (1981) used a multiple biopsy technique to examine the uterine cavities of 22 women using IUDs. In five women, wearing a tailless IUD, the uterus was sterile, and in 15 of 17 women wearing a tailed device, bacteria were found in the uterus but they had not reached the fundus. Duration of IUD use ranged from $7\frac{1}{2}$ months to 9 years. The surface bacterial counts showed a diminishing number of bacteria in the uterine cavity and no differences between monofilamentous and multifilamentous tails. No PID infection was found. The authors suggest that the bacterial colonization is usually harmless because of the small number of bacteria, the failure of the bacteria to reach the fundus, and local defense mechanisms.

Neisseria gonorrhoeae

Neisseria gonorrhoeae has been isolated from the cervices of from 10% to 70% of women with salpingitis (Curran, 1979; Eschenbach and Holmes, 1979). The wide span of results may be accounted for by differences in the prevalence of cervical gonorrhea in various countries, by different virulence of gonococci in various parts of the world, by differences in the racial composition of socioeconomic status in the populations studied (Holmes *et al.*, 1980) and by probable differences in techniques used at various centers for recovering and cultivating gonococci, which are highly sensitive to changes in the environment.

Berger *et al.* (1975) found among 2005 women attending the Family Planning Clinic in Shreveport, Louisiana (USA), gonorrheal culture in 11.5% of oral contraceptive (OC) users, in 9.9% of IUD users, and in 7.8%

of controls (RR for IUD users was 1.3, for OC users 1.5). The differences were not significant. Two studies (Ryden *et al.*, 1979 and McCormack *et al.*, 1977) found a higher prevalence of gonococci in IUD users than in non-users while four other studies found that in IUD users, non-gonococcal PID was more frequent than gonococcal infections (Eschenbach *et al.*, 1977; Osser *et al.*, 1980; Westrom *et al.*, 1976; Paavonen and Vesterinem, 1980). Westrom *et al.* (1976) did not find a difference in the prevalence of PID between users of polyethylene and copper IUDs.

When analyzing 274 IUDs removed for PID, Nilsson *et al.* (1981) found that positive cultures of *Neisseria gonorrhoeae* clearly correlated with the severity of the inflammatory disease.

Chlamydia

Since 1975, when Eschenbach *et al.* first mentioned it in connection with PID, chlamydia has been gaining reputation as one of the most frequent PID agents. In women with PID, it has been found in 20–36% (Eschenbach *et al.*, 1975; Mardh *et al.*, 1977), while it was found in 3–13% of PID-free women.

Prevalence of chlamydia in users of various contraceptive methods was discussed by Mardh *et al.* (1977). In 24 IUD users with PID, they cultured chlamydia from the cervix in 38% and, in 11 OC users with PID, 54%. The article does not provide a comparison with women not using contraceptives. Hren-Vencelj (1980) isolated chlamydia in two of 29 IUD users, in one of 43 OC users, and in nine of 122 non-users. The difference in the prevalence of chlamydia in the three groups was not significant. The preliminary data of the Ljubljana PID study on the prevalence of chlamydia in women hospitalized for PID, by type of contraceptive, are given in Table 5.8 (Kozuh-Novak *et al.*, 1983).

Chlamydia was found in 20% of women with PID and in 14% of controls. Chlamydia was more frequent in both IUD and OC users with PID than in PID-free contraceptive users (RR = 1.8 and 1.7, respectively). In non-users, the difference between PID and PID-free women is smaller (RR = 1.3). Chlamydia was significantly more frequent in IUD users than

Table 5.8 *Chlamydia trachomatis* in women with PID and in controls, by the type of contraceptive

Contraceptive	PID		No PID	
	Chl +	*Chl −*	*Chl +*	*Chl −*
None	9	55	5	39
OC	11	30	6	28
IUD	13	34	4	19
Barrier methods	2	15	1	3
Others	4	21	1	16
Total	39	155	17	105

in non-users of contraceptives. Similar results were obtained when comparing OC users with PID and non-users with PID ($RR = 2.2$). But in PID-free women, in spite of a higher prevalence of chlamydia in both IUD and OC users, the differences are not significant ($RR = 1.6$ for both types of contraceptives).

Actinomyces

Gupta *et al.* (1976) have reported actinomyces-like organisms in cervical smears of IUD users. Curtis and Pine (1981) examined 50 women and found actinomyces in the mucus from the external cervical os in 36%. Actinomyces was found in 44% of 18 IUD users and in 27% of 30 non-users. The difference was not significant.

Aubert *et al.* (1980) searched for actinomyces in 763 women whose IUD was removed for unspecified medical reasons. In the endometrial tissue, actinomyces was found in 3.14%. The women had used an IUD for 24-122 months (with the average duration of 62 months).

In women with PID, actinomyces is rare. In the past few years, 83 cases of actinomycosis-related PID have been reported among women using IUDs or pessaries. The data suggest that actinomycosis infections of the female genital tract among IUD users increase with duration of use (Edelman *et al.*, 1982). The data do not suggest an association between the duration of IUD use and the severity of infection.

It has been suggested that when actinomyces-like organisms are found in the cervical smear, the IUD should be removed (IPPF-IMAP, 1981). We believe, however, that before accepting this statement, more data should be collected pertaining to the incidence of PID in those women.

DISCUSSION

Most epidemiologic studies pertaining to a correlation between PID and IUD use have been based on the clinical diagnosis of PID. Jacobson and Westrom (1969), however, were able to confirm the accuracy of clinical diagnoses by means of laparoscopy in only 65% of 814 women. Similarly, Chaparro *et al.* (1978) confirmed the diagnosis in 46% of laparoscopically rediagnosed cases. Thus, the validity of results in most epidemiologic studies is limited, and the validity of laparoscopy is also open to question. The authors of the studies cited above performed laparoscopies only in hospitalized patients. Practicing gynecologists are mainly concerned with early diagnosis to prevent complications. In mild infections, laparoscopy seems too invasive and is ethically questionable, a consideration supported by the striking finding of Holmes *et al.* (1980) that primary salpingitis can rarely be confirmed laparoscopically in women who do not have increased leukocytes in the vaginal fluid and/or a proven sexually transmitted infection. Therefore, it is our belief that studies of mild infections, which are most frequent and easiest to prevent, should continue to be based on clinical and laboratory diagnostic procedures.

Future studies on PID in IUD users should address improved means of detecting bacterial strains in the cervical canal, and diagnosing silent subacute or chronic pelvic infections. Studies should examine the relationship between long-term usage of the IUD, as well as intermenstrual spotting or bleeding and PID, and should explore the interaction between various bacteria and immunoprotective systems of the genital tract.

References

Adams, D.B., Rose-Gold, A. and Burt, A.D. (1978). Rise in female-initiated sexual activity at ovulation and its suppression by oral contraceptives. *N. Engl. J. Med.*, **299**, 1145-50

Aubert, J.M., Gobeaux-Castadot, M.J. and Boria, M.C. (1980). Actinomyces in the endometrium of IUD users. *Contraception*, **21**, 577-83

Berger, G.S., Keith, L. and Moss, W. (1975). Prevalence of gonorrhoea among women using methods of contraception. *Br. J. Vener. Dis.*, **51**, 307-9

Burkman, R.T. and The Women's Health Study (1981). Association between intrauterine device and pelvic inflammatory disease. *Obstet. Gynecol.*, **57**, 269-76

Chaparro, M.V., Ghosh, S., Nashed, A. and Poliak, A. (1978). Laparoscopy for the confirmation and prognostic evaluation of pelvic inflammatory disease. *Int. J. Gynaecol. Obstet.*, **15**, 307-9

Curran, J.W. (1979). Management of gonococcal pelvic inflammatory disease. *Sex. Transm. Dis. (Suppl.)*, **6**, 174-80

Curtis, E.M. and Pine, L. (1981). Actinomyces in the vaginas of women with and without intrauterine contraceptive devices. *Am. J. Obstet. Gynecol.*, **140**, 880-4

Danev, M. and Kozuh-Novak, M. (1983). Register on complications in IUD users requiring hospital treatment. *Report to the Committee for Health and Social Security of Slovenia, Ljubljana*

Edelman, D.A., Berger, G.S. and Keith, L. (1982). The use of IUDs and their relationship to pelvic inflammatory disease: a review of epidemiologic and clinical studies. *Curr. Prob. Obstet. Gynecol.*, **6**, 1

Eschenbach, D.A. (1980). Epidemiology and diagnosis of acute pelvic inflammatory disease. *Obstet. Gynecol.*, **55** (Suppl.), 142S-535S

Eschenbach, D.A., Buchanan, T.M., Pollock, H.M. *et al.* (1975). Polymicrobial etiology of acute pelvic inflammatory disease. *N. Engl. J. Med.*, **293**, 166-71

Eschenbach, D.A., Harnisch, J.P. and Holmes, K.K. (1977). Pathogenesis of acute pelvic inflammatory disease: role of contraception and other risk factors. *Am. J. Obstet. Gynecol.*, **128**, 838-50

Eschenbach, D.A. and Holmes, K.K. (1979). The etiology of acute pelvic inflammatory disease. *Sex. Transm. Dis.*, **6**, 224-7

Faulkner, W.L. and Ory, H.W. (1976). Intrauterine devices and acute pelvic inflammatory disease. *J. Am. Med. Assoc.*, **235**, 1851-3

Goldacre, M.J., Watt, B., London, N. *et al.* (1979). Vaginal microbial flora in normal young women. *Br. Med. J.*, **1**, 1550-5

Gupta, P.K., Hollander, D.H. and Frost, J.K. (1976). Actinomyces in cervicovaginal smears: an association with IUD usage. *Acta Cytol.*, **20**, 295-7

Holmes, K.K., Eschenbach, D.A. and Knapp, J.S. (1980). Salpingitis: overview of etiology and epidemiology. *Am. J. Obstet. Gynecol.*, **138**, 893-900

Hren-Vencelj, H. (1980). The role of *chlamydia trachomatis* in human pathology. *Report to the Research Foundation of Slovenia, Ljubljana*

IPPF-IMAP (1981). Statement on intrauterine devices. *IPPF Med. Bull.*, **15**, 1

Jacobson, L. and Westrom, L. (1969). Objectivized diagnosis of acute pelvic inflammatory disease. *Am. J. Obstet. Gynecol.*, **105**, 1088-98

Jones, M.C., Buschmann, B.O., Dowling, E.A. *et al.* (1979). The prevalence of actinomyces-like organisms found in cervicovaginal smears of 300 IUD wearers. *Acta Cytol.*, **23**, 282

Kaufman, D., Shapiro, S., Rosenberg, L., Monson, R.R., Miettinen, O.S., Stolley, P.D. and

BIOMEDICAL ASPECTS OF IUDs

Slone, D. (1980). Intrauterine contraceptive device use and pelvic inflammatory disease. *Am. J. Obstet. Gynecol.*, **136**, 159-62

Kozuh-Novak, M. and Andolsek, L. (1980). Pregnancy rate after longer use of two copper IUDs. *Contracept. Deliv. Syst.*, **1**, 95

Kozuh-Novak, M. and Andolsek, L. (1982). Risk factors for PID among IUD users. Paper presented at *International Symposium on Reproductive Care*, October 10-15, 1982, Maui, Hawaii, USA. *Contracept. Deliv. Syst.*, **3**, Abstract 203

Kozuh-Novak, M., Andolsek, L., Kunej, Z., Hren, H. and Gubina, M. (1983). Ljubljana PID study. *Preliminary report to the Research Foundation of Slovenia, Ljubljana*

Lippes, J. (1975). The loop after ten years. In Hefnawi, F. and Segal, S.I. (eds.) *Analysis of Intrauterine Contraception.* p. 225. (Amsterdam: North-Holland Publishing Company)

Luukkainen, T., Nielsen, N.C., Nygren, K.G. and Pyorala, T. (1979). Nulliparous women, IUD and pelvic infection. *Ann. Clinic. Res.*, **11**, 121-4

McCormack, W.M., Johnson, K., Stumacher, R.J. *et al.* (1977). Clinical spectrum of gonococcal infection in women. *Lancet*, **1**, 1182 5

Maqueo, M.T., Calderon, J.J. and Guerra, A.Z. (1979). Salpingitis associated with the presence of nonmedicated IUDs. *Contraception*, **19**, 539-42

Mardh, P.A., Ripa, T., Svensson, L. and Westrom, L. (1977). *Chlamydia trachomatis* infection in patients with acute salpingitis. *N. Engl. J. Med.*, **296**, 1377-9

Nilsson, C.G., Vartiainen, E. and Widholm, O. (1981). Bacterial cultures from intrauterine devices removed from patients with pelvic inflammatory disease. *Acta Obstet. Gynecol. Scand.*, **60**, 563-6

Odevald, E. (1976). The biophysical aspects of cervical mucus. In Jordan, J.A. and Singer, A. (eds.) *The Cervix.* p. 155. (London: Saunders)

Osser, S., Liedholm, P., Gullberg, B. *et al.* (1980). Risk of pelvic inflammatory disease among intrauterine device users irrespective of previous pregnancy. *Lancet*, **2**, 386-8

Paavonen, J. and Vesterinem, E. (1980). Intrauterine contraceptive device use in patients with acute salpingitis. *Contraception*, **22**, 107-14

Parrier, B.G.A., Sparks, R.A., Watt, P.J. and Elstein, M. (1979). *In vitro* study of the possible role of the intrauterine contraceptive tail in ascending infection of the genital tract. *Br. J. Obstet. Gynaecol.*, **86**, 374-8

Phaosavaski, S., Vivanichakul, B., Rienprayura, D. *et al.* (1975). Pelvic inflammatory disease in contraceptive acceptors disclosed at transvaginal tubal sterilization. In Hefnawi, F. and Segal, S.I. (eds.) *Analysis of Intrauterine Contraception.* p.397. (Amsterdam, North-Holland)

Ryden, G., Fahraeus, L., Molin, L. *et al.* (1979). Do contraceptives influence the incidence of acute pelvic inflammatory disease in women with gonorrhea? *Contraception*, **20**, 149-57

Senanayake, P. and Kramer, D.G. (1980). Contraception and the etiology of pelvic inflammatory disease: new perspectives. *Am. J. Obstet. Gynecol.*, **138**, 852-60

Sparks, R.A., Parrier, B., Watt, P.J. and Elstein, M. (1981). Bacteriological colonisation of uterine cavity: role of tailed intrauterine device. *Br. Med. J.*, **282**, 1189-91

Targum, S.D. and Wright, N.H. (1974). Association of the intrauterine device and pelvic inflammatory disease: a retrospective study. *Am. J. Epidemiol.*, **100**, 262

Vessey, M.P., Yeates, D., Flavel, R. *et al.* (1981). Pelvic inflammatory disease and the intrauterine device: findings in a large cohort study. *Br. Med. J.*, **14**, 855-7

Watt, B., Goldacre, M.J., Loudon, N., Annat, D.J., Harris, R.I. and Vessey, M.P. (1981). Prevalence of bacteria in the vagina of normal young women. *Br. J. Obstet. Gynecol.*, **88**, 588-95

Westrom, L., Bengtsson, L.P. and Mardh, P.A. (1976). The risk of pelvic inflammatory disease in women using intrauterine contraceptive devices as compared to non-users. *Lancet*, **1**, 221-4

World Health Organization (1982). Interval IUD insertion in parous women: a randomized multicentre comparative trial of the Lippes Loop D, T Cu 220C and the Copper 7. *Contraception*, **26**, 1-22

Wright, N.H. and Laemmle, P. (1968). Acute pelvic inflammatory disease in an indigent population. *Am. J. Obstet. Gynecol.*, **101**, 979-90

Zipper, J., Medel, M., Osorio, A., Goldsmith, A. and Edelman, D. (1976). Long-term use effectiveness of the Cu-7-200 IUD. *Int. J. Gynecol. Obstet.*, **14**, 142-4

6
IUD complications

B. W. SIMCOCK

INTRODUCTION

Many of the complications associated with intrauterine devices (IUDs) can be managed on an outpatient basis provided the physician is aware of conditions that require hospitalization. In some urban areas of developed countries, patients may be hospitalized unnecessarily for IUD-related problems. On the other hand, in rural areas of developing countries, hospitalization for serious IUD complications may be delayed as a result of attitudinal and economic factors. This chapter describes IUD complications relative to the need for hospitalization.

MENOMETRORRHAGIA

Abnormal uterine bleeding is the most common IUD complication. Various medications have been proposed to control this problem with inconclusive results. Removal of the device generally ameliorates the abnormal bleeding pattern and/or excessive menstrual loss. This is usually accomplished in the physician's office. However, should excessive bleeding continue following IUD removal, the patient should be hospitalized for a diagnostic dilatation and curettage. Huggins (1981) reviewed 545 cases of bleeding associated with IUD use that required hospitalization. In 49 women the condition required blood transfusion. Huggins compared these cases to 3453 controls and reported no significant association between IUD use and hospitalization for unexplained vaginal bleeding.

PELVIC INFLAMMATORY DISEASE (PID)

An epidemic rise in the incidence of PID has been noted in many developed countries since the late 1960s. In 1974, for instance, 874161 cases of gonorrhea were reported in the US, probably accounting for a large proportion of PID cases. Westrom *et al.* (1976) found, however, that although the rate of PID continued to increase in Sweden, the rate of gonococcal salpingitis decreased indicating that non-gonococcal infections may have become a more significant factor in the causation of PID. A causative relationship between IUD use and pelvic inflammatory disease has been demonstrated by several investigators (Burkman, 1981; Eschenbach and Holmes, 1975; Eschenbach *et al.*, 1977; Faulkner and Ory, 1976; Kaufman *et al.*, 1980; Ory, 1978; Osser *et al.*, 1980; Targum and Wright, 1974; Vessey *et al.*, 1981; Westrom *et al.*, 1976). Several factors were reported to increase the risk for PID in IUD users: socioeconomic status, number of sexual partners, previous history of salpingitis (Edelman and Berger 1980; Flesh *et al.*, 1979), age (Booth *et al.*, 1980), parity (Eschenbach *et al.*, 1977; Westrom *et al.*, 1976), duration of IUD use (Kaufman *et al.*, 1980) and the presence of *actinomyces israelii* in cytologic samples from the genital tract (Burkman *et al.*, 1982; Drew, 1981; Fulton *et al.*, 1981). Barwin *et al.* (1978) found that incidence of PID in the low socioeconomic group was 2–5 times higher than in a group of more privileged patients. Booth *et al.* (1980) studied the rate of PID in nulliparous women using the copper-7 IUD and found that women in the 16–19 age-group had more than ten times the risk of women in the 30–49 age-group. The rate of PID was greatest in the first six months of use. The effect of copper-bearing IUDs on lowering the rate of PID was confirmed by some investigators (Buckingham *et al.*, 1976; Kaufman *et al.*, 1980) and denied by others (Ory, 1978; Paavonen and Vesterinem, 1980).

It should be noted however, that the diagnosis of PID on clinical grounds is unreliable (Buckingham *et al.*, 1976; Jacobson and Westrom, 1969) and that the selection of patients in case-controlled studies is often subject to unavoidable bias (Gray, 1980). For instance, in many studies the rate of PID in IUD users is compared to that of women using oral contraceptives, a method generally recognized as protecting its users against PID. Furthermore, in other studies reporting high PID rates with IUD users, laparoscopic confirmation of the diagnosis was not obtained. When laparoscopy was performed in patients suspected of having PID many were found to have conditions other than PID (Jacobson and Westrom, 1969).

Patients suspected of having mild PID can be treated with antibiotics in the physician's office. Others suspected of having severe PID should be hospitalized, treated with intravenous antibiotic therapy pending laparoscopic confirmation (Herschey, 1980) (which is frequently required) and monitored (Spaulding *et al.*, 1979) with leukocytic counts, sedimentation rate and ultrasonography. Appropriate bacteriological cultures should be taken. Patients with pelvic and/or tubo-ovarian abscesses are treated surgically. Aggressive management is recommended in order to minimize the occurrence of serious complications (Edelman and Berger, 1980; Kum and Charles, 1979; Maloy *et al.*, 1981; Onsrud, 1980). Although removal of the IUD is usually incorporated in the management, it has been reported that such a practice does not influence the outcome (Larsson *et al.*, 1979). Patients with one or more risk factors should be advised to seek an alternative method of contraception.

THE LOST IUD

In patients presenting with a missing IUD string one of the following events has taken place:

(1) The IUD has been expelled.
(2) The device is concealed within the uterine cavity.
(3) The device has perforated the uterine wall and/or migrated into the peritoneal cavity.

Expulsion should be confirmed by ultrasonography (Gentile and Siegler, 1977; McArdle, 1978) or X-rays (Gentile and Siegler, 1977). The patient may be evaluated in the consulting room by probing the uterine cavity with a sterile sound in order to locate the device. The IUD may be concealed within the uterus if the string is retracted into the cavity and lost from view. Once uterine presence of the IUD is confirmed, it may be possible to draw the string down through the cervical canal with various instruments and much operator skill, thus avoiding the need for hospitalization. Rao (1978), Zakin et al. (1981), and Gentile and Siegler (1977) have written excellent reviews on this subject.

Should attempts to retrieve the string meet with no success then hospital admission is required for removal of the device under general or local anesthesia. Reviewing the records in my hospital, I found 51 admissions for this purpose over a 2-year period. In six of the women, the IUD had perforated the uterus. One of these women became pregnant following the perforation. Valle et al. (1977) used hysteroscopy to retrieve a 'lost' IUD thread in a series of 91 women. They located and removed the IUD in 78 patients, discovered that the device had translocated into the abdominal cavity in six patients and did not find the IUD in 13 patients, indicating that unnoticed expulsion had occurred. In a similar study of a smaller series of 23 patients, Gupta et al. (1977) successfully removed 21 IUDs (with retracted or missing threads), and were able to confirm expulsion in one woman and translocation of the device in another.

The third possible event is perforation of the uterine wall, and migration or translocation of the device, intraperitoneally, or retroperitoneally below the pouch of Douglas, or in the anterior vesical pouch. In such cases, the nature of the device affects the outcome. Inert IUDs were reported to wander freely about the peritoneal cavity without showing a tendency to form adhesions (Lippes, 1976). It was suggested that inert IUDs that have translocated into the peritoneal cavity present no risk to the patient and therefore should not be removed (Lippes, 1976). It should be noted, however, that large bowel perforation by 'inert' translocated devices, namely the Lippes loop and Dalkon Shield have occurred resulting in serious problems (Kirkpatrick et al., 1975). It is generally agreed that all closed ring devices and copper-containing devices should be removed because of the danger of bowel obstruction and the formation of dense vascular adhesions that characteristically (and rapidly) develop around a copper device.

Laparoscopy is useful for removing intra-abdominal devices, particularly those of the inert type (McKenna and Mylotte, 1982; Osborne and Bennett,

1978; Pearce, 1976). In one study reporting 67 translocations over 6 years, nearly all of the inert devices were retrieved laparoscopically but only about 44% of the copper devices were removed by this method (McKenna and Mylotte, 1982).

The risk of IUD perforation depends upon many factors, including the type of device and introducer (Edelman and Berger, 1980), skill of the provider (Hall, 1967), age and parity of the patient, interval since last delivery or abortion, and condition of uterine wall (Edelman and Berger, 1980). For instance 87% of translocations reported in one study arose from postpartum or postabortal insertions (McKenna and Mylotte, 1982). Ratnam and Tow (1970) reported that the incidence of uterine perforations with IUDs varied between 0.5 and 9.0 per 1000 insertions.

IUD perforations may present with unusual complaints. In one bizarre case, a woman complained of feeling her IUD strings emerging per rectum and was subsequently found to have suffered a posterior perforation through a retroverted uterus into the sigmoid colon (Beard, 1981). Other investigators reported two cases of stricture of the mid-rectum following extensive pelvic cellulitis due to the use of IUDs (Rogers and Hughes, 1982) and two cases of bowel perforations with copper devices (Key and Kreutner, 1980).

A device may be partially outside of the uterine cavity with its string still visible at the uterine external os. The perforated portion of the device may become embedded into adjoining bowel wall. Hence, forceful removal of a device is unwise as it may tear the bowel wall leading to severe sepsis, or pelvic abscess.

Many hospitalizations could be prevented simply by knowing the type of IUD the patient is wearing. Two women wearing IUDs were admitted to an Australian hospital after the doctor had been unable to find a string on inspection. The women had Graafenberg rings which have no retrieval string. Normally, removal of a Graafenberg ring is a simple outpatient procedure, using a ring hook remover.

ECTOPIC PREGNANCY

Since 1970, there has been a dramatic increase in the incidence of ectopic pregnancy. In the US, between 1965 and 1977, the rate trebled (Ory, 1981). The possible reasons for this increased rate include: use of the IUD, the progestogen-only pill, previous tubal surgery (tubal ligation, tubal re-anastomosis) and history of prior PID (Weekes and Hutchins, 1976). PID was reported to be the principal cause accounting for the increased incidence of ectopic pregnancy, accounting for 69% of the cases in one study (Weekes and Hutchins, 1976) and 35% in another (Pagano, 1981). 8.2% of the patients in the first study and 14% of the patients in the second study were using an IUD at the time. Another study investigating the relationship between PID, IUD and ectopic pregnancy concluded that PID, regardless of etiology, was the principal cause of ectopic pregnancy and that the IUD *per se* is probably not a causal factor in ectopic pregnancy (Hallatt, 1976).

In the USA, analysis of the National Hospital Discharge Survey figures indicated that the IUD is not a major factor contributing to the marked rise in the rate of ectopic pregnancy (Sivin, 1979). Another epidemiologic study did not find an association between ectopic pregnancy and pelvic infection (Beral, 1975). Thus, the factors involved in the recent rise of ectopic pregnancy are still debatable.

The absolute risk for ectopic pregnancy among IUD users is fairly constant throughout the duration of use at 1.2 per 1000 women per year (Vessey, 1979), and does not appear to be affected by parity (Malhotra and Chaundhury, 1982). However, the risk may be greater for women using progestogen IUDs as compared with women using copper or inert devices, as reported by Snowden (1977). Diaz *et al.* (1980) in a comparative study of various progestogen-releasing IUDs, also found that five of 12 pregnancies occurring with these IUDs were ectopic compared with none out of ten pregnancies occurring in the control copper IUD group.

Hallatt (1982) found that of 25 ovarian ectopic pregnancies, 20% were associated with IUD use. Most patients did not suspect they were pregnant; amenorrhea was present in only 17% of tubal pregnancies and 16% of ovarian pregnancies. Hallatt (1976) recommends that ectopic pregnancy should be suspected in any patient with an IUD who has irregular bleeding and abdominal pain; in 75% of patients in his study the diagnosis was not made at the first examination. Apparently, the IUD does prevent tubal or ovarian ectopic pregnancies efficiently, as its principal action is on the endometrium.

The management of ectopic pregnancy associated with IUD use rests on having a high incidence of suspicion especially with progestogen devices and on instituting appropriate diagnostic procedures including pregnancy tests, ultrasonography and laparoscopy. Conservative surgical management is usually indicated.

INTRAUTERINE PREGNANCY

Although there is no evidence of a teratogenic effect exerted by any IUD upon a developing fetus, many physicians advise their pregnant IUD patients to terminate the pregnancy. Studies of tissues obtained from 394 women who spontaneously aborted showed that there is a lower incidence of embryonic abnormalities in women using IUDs (21%) than in women using no contraception (44%) (Poland, 1970) I have found that many women, feeling negatively motivated to continue a pregnancy that they have taken considerable steps to prevent, request termination despite reassurances about the normality of the conceptus.

On the other hand, if the IUD is left *in situ* the danger of spontaneous abortion is high. Investigators report a rate of abortion of around 55% which is about three times the normal rate (Lewit, 1970; Tatum *et al.*, 1976; Vessey *et al.*, 1976). Currently, it is standard practice to remove the IUD from a pregnant uterus at the earliest opportunity, if the woman elects to continue with the pregnancy. Studies have shown that the spontaneous abortion rate diminishes after the removal of the IUD but not quite to normal levels of 13–18% (Vessey *et al.*, 1976). Alvior (1973) reported a 29% abortion rate in 81 women from whom a Lippes Loop was removed. Under similar circumstances, Tatum *et al.* (1976) found an even lower abortion rate of 20.3% with the Copper T IUD.

Women who elect to keep the IUD during pregnancy have an increased risk for developing septic abortion. In the 2 years from 1972 to 1974, 50 maternal deaths due to septic abortion were reported: 17 of them with an IUD *in situ* (13 Dalkon Shield, three Lippes Loop and one Saf-T-Coil) (Cates, 1977). The risk of death from septic abortion was 14.8 per 100 000 women with an IUD as compared to 0.28 per 100 000 women without an IUD. Although this rate may have been affected by a bias, IUD septic abortions may have been over-reported and non-IUD septic abortions under-reported, nevertheless the difference is significant. For 2 or 3 years after 1974, no IUD-related deaths were reported even though IUDs continued to be used. This may have been due to recommendations issued by IUD manufacturers that IUDs should be removed from all women when a pregnancy occurred.

The rate of septic abortion and other pregnancy complications was reported to be greater for the Dalkon Shield than for other IUDs (Kahn and Tyler, 1976). The multifilament tail of the Dalkon Shield was thought by some (Tatum *et al.*, 1975) to provide a potential reservoir for bacteria as it was drawn up into the endometrial cavity with the onset of pregnancy. The rate of septic abortion for IUDs other than the Dalkon Shield may not be significantly different from the rate among women who conceive while using other contraceptive methods or no methods. In one study, 58 of 115 abortions occurred in women using IUDs, the remaining 57 abortions occurred in women using other methods. Sepsis was reported in only six women: four in the IUD group and two in the other group (Williams *et al.*, 1975).

Women who carry an IUD during pregnancy must be instructed to notify their physicians immediately if bleeding or fever occurs. Septic abortion with an IUD in place is a life-threatening complication which requires aggressive inpatient hospital management.

CONCLUSION

The management of IUD-related problems is an area where judgement, skill and diagnostic ability are important and, if guidelines are laid down and adhered to, then the use of IUDs would not arouse fear and apprehension in the minds of many women.

References

Alvior, G. T., (1973). Pregnancy outcome with removal of intrauterine device. *Obstet. Gynecol.*, **41**, 894–6

Barwin, B. N., Tuttle S. and Jolly, E. E. (1978). The intrauterine contraceptive device. *Can. Med. Assoc. J.*, **118**, 53–8

Beard, R. J. (1981). Unusual presentation of translocated IUD. *Lancet*, **1**, 837

Beral, V. (1975). An epidemiological study of recent trends in ectopic pregnancy. *Br. J. Obstet. Gynaecol.*, **82**, 775 82

Booth, M., Beral, V. and Guillebaud. J. (1980). Effect of age on pelvic inflammatory disease in nulliparous women using a copper-7 intrauterine contraceptive device. *Br. Med. J.*, **281**, 114–5

Buckingham, M. S., Sparks, R. A., Watt, P. J. and Elstein, M. (1976). Pelvic infection and intrauterine devices. *Br. Med. J.*, **2**, 942 3

Burkman, R. T. (1981). Association between intrauterine device and pelvic inflammatory disease. *Obstet. Gynecol.*, **57**, 269 76

Burkman, R. T., Schlesselman, S., McCaffrey, L., Gupta, P. K. and Spence, M. (1982). The relationship of genital tract actinomycetes and the development of pelvic inflammatory disease. *Am. J. Obstet. Gynecol.*, **143**, 585 9

Cates, W. (1977). Publicity and the public health: the elimination of IUD-related abortion deaths. *Fam. Plann. Persp.*, **9**, 138 40

Diaz, S. *et al.* (1980). Ectopic pregnancies associated with low dose progestogen-releasing IUDs. *Contraception*, **22**, 259 69

Drew, N. C. (1981) Genital and pelvic actinomycosis. *Br. J. Obstet. Gynaecol.*, **88**, 776-7

Edelman, D. A. and Berger, G. S. (1980). Contraceptive practice and tubo-ovarian abscess. *Am. J. Obstet. Gynecol.*, **138**, 541 4

Eschenbach, D. A., Harnisch, J. P. and Holmes, K. K., (1977). Pathogenesis of acute pelvic inflammatory disease; role of contraception and other risk factors. *Am. J. Obstet. Gynecol.*, **128**, 838-50

Eschenbach, D. A. and Holmes, K. K. (1975). Acute pelvic inflammatory disease: current concepts of pathogenesis, etiology and management. *Clin. Obstet. Gynecol.*, **18**, 35-56

Faulkner, W. L. and Ory, H. W. (1976). Intrauterine devices and acute pelvic inflammatory disease. *J. Am. Med. Assoc.*, **235**, 1851 3

Flesh, G., Weiner, J. M., Corlett, R. C., Boice, C., Mishell, D. R. and Wolf, R. M. (1979). The intrauterine device and acute salpingitis: a multi-factor analysis. *Am. J. Obstet. Gynecol.*, **135**, 402 8

Fulton, I. C., Paterson, W. G. and Crucioli, V. (1981). Pelvic actinomycosis causing ureteric obstruction. *Br. J. Obstet. Gynaecol.*, **88**, 1044-50

Gentile, G. P. and Siegler, A. M. (1977). The missing or misplaced intrauterine device. *Obstet. Gynaecol. Survey*, **32**, 627 41

Gray, R. H. (1980). Letter. *Lancet*, **1**, 718

Gupta, I., Devi, P. K. and Gupta, A. N. (1977). Hysteroscopic removal of intrauterine contraceptive devices with missing threads. *Ind. J. Med. Res.*, **65**, 661-3

Hall, R. E. (1967). A reappraisal of IUDs. Prompted by the delayed discovery of uterine perforations. *Am. J. Obstet. Gynecol.*, **99**, 808

Hallatt, J. G. (1976). Ectopic pregnancy associated with the intrauterine device: a study of seventy cases. *Am. J. Obstet. Gynecol.*, **125**, 754 8

Hallatt, J. G. (1982). Primary ovarian pregnancy: a report of 25 cases. *Am. J. Obstet. Gynecol.*, **143**, 55-60

Herschey, D. W. (1980). Management of a patient with an intrauterine device and a unilateral adnexal mass. *J. Reprod. Med.*, **25**, 75 8

Huggins, G. R. (1981). IUD use and unexplained vaginal bleeding. *Obstet. Gynecol.*, **58**, 409-16

Jacobson, L. and Westrom. L. (1969). Objectivized diagnosis of acute pelvic inflammatory disease. *Am. J. Obstet. Gynecol.*, **105**, 1088-98

Kahn, H. S. and Tyler, C. W. (1976). An association between the Dalkon Shield and complicated pregnancies among women hospitalized for intrauterine contraceptive device-related disorders. *Am. J. Obstet. Gynecol.*, **125**, 83 6

Kaufman, D. W. *et al.* (1980). Intrauterine contraceptive device use and pelvic inflammatory disease. *Am. J. Obstet. Gynecol.*, **136**, 159 62

Key, T. C. and Kreutner, A. K. (1980). Case reports gastrointestinal complications of modern intrauterine devices. *Obstet. Gynecol.*, **55**, 239-44

Kirkpatrick, D., Schneider, J. and Paterson, E. P. (1975). Large bowel perforation by intrauterine devices. *Obstet. Gynecol.*, **46**, 610 12

Kum, N. and Charles, D. (1979). Cerebral abscess associated with an intrauterine contraceptive device. *Obstet. Gynecol.*, **54**, 375 8

Larsson, B., Hagstrom, B., Viberg, L., Anker, C., Hamberger, L. and Lindhe, B. A. (1979). Low risk of pelvic inflammatory disease in young never-pregnant women using Gravigard R. *Contraception*, **20**, 291-5

Lewit, S. (1970). Outcome of pregnancies with intrauterine devices. *Contraception*, **2**, 47-53

Lippes, J. (1976). Letter. *J. Am. Med. Assoc.*, **235**, 1001

McArdle, C. (1978). Ultrasonic localization of missing intrauterine contraceptive devices. *Obstet. Gynecol.*, **51**, 330-3

McKenna, P. J. and Mylotte, M. J. (1982). Laparoscopic removal of translocated intrauterine contraceptive devices. *Br. J. Obstet. Gynaecol.*, **89**, 163-5

Malhotra, N. and Chaundhury, R. (1982). Current status of IUDs. II. Intrauterine devices and pelvic inflammatory disease and ectopic pregnancy. *Obstet. Gynecol. Survey*, **37**, 1-8

Maloy, A. L., Meier, F. A. and Karl, R. C. (1981). Fatal peritonitis following IUD-associated salpingitis. *Obstet. Gynecol.*, **58**, 397-8

Onsrud, M. (1980). Perihepatitis in pelvic inflammatory disease—association with intrauterine contraception. *Acta Obstet. Gynecol. Scand.*, **55**, 69-71

Ory, H. W. (1978). A review of the association between the intrauterine device and acute pelvic inflammatory disease. *J. Reprod. Med.*, **20**, 200-4

Ory, H. W. (1981). Ectopic pregnancy and intrauterine devices: new perspectives. *Obstet. Gynecol.*, **57**, 137-44

Osborne, J. L. and Bennett, M. J. (1978). Removal of intra-abdominal intrauterine contraceptive device. *Br. J. Obstet. Gynaecol.*, **85**, 868-71

Osser, S., Liedholm, P. and Sjoberg, N. D. (1980). Risk of pelvic inflammatory disease among intrauterine device users irrespective of previous pregnancy. *Lancet*, **1**, 386; *Am. J. Obstet. Gynecol*, **138**, (7 Pt 2), 864-7

Paavonen, J. and Vesterinem, E. (1980). Intrauterine device use in patients with acute salpingitis. *Contraception*, **22**, 107-14

Pagano, R. (1981). Ectopic pregnancy: a 7 year survey. *Med. J. Aust.*, **2**, 586-8

Pearce, D. J. (1976). Laparoscopic removal of IUDs from the abdomen. Letter. *Br. Med. J.*, **1**, 1017

Poland, B. (1970). Conception control and embryonic development. *Am. J. Obstet. Gynecol.*, **106**, 365-8

Rao, R. P. (1978). Lost intrauterine devices and their localization. *J. Reprod. Med.*, **20**, 195-9

Ratnam, S. and Tow, S. H. (1970). Translocation of the loop. In Zatuchni, G. I. (ed.) *Post partum Family Planning. A Report on the International Program*. (New York: McGraw-Hill)

Rogers, K. and Hughes, L. E. (1982). Rectal strictures associated with the intrauterine contraceptive device. *Br. J. Surg.*, **69**, 151-2

Sivin, I. (1979). Copper T use and ectopic pregnancy rates in the U.S. *Contraception*, **19**, 151-73

Snowden, R. (1977). The Progestasert and ectopic pregnancy. *Br. Med. J.*, **2**, 1600-1

Spaulding, L. B., Gelman, S. R., Wood, S. D. and Monif, G. R. (1979). The role of ultrasonography in the management of endometritis/salpingitis/peritonitis. *Obstet. Gynecol.* **53**, 442-6

Targum, S. D. and Wright, N. H. (1974). Association of the intrauterine device and pelvic inflammatory disease: a retrospective pilot study. *Am. J. Epidem.*, **100**, 262-71

Tatum, H. J., Schmidt, F. H., Phillips, D., McCarty, M. and O'Leary, W. M. (1975). The Dalkon Shield controversy: structural and bacteriological studies of IUD tails. *J. Am. Med. Assoc.*, **231**, 711-17

Tatum, H., Schmidt, E. H. and Jain, A. K. (1976). Management and outcome of pregnancies associated with Copper T IUD. *Am. J. Obstet. Gynecol.*, **7**, 869-79

Valle, R. F., Sciarra, J. J. and Freeman, D. W. (1977). Hysteroscopic removal of intrauterine devices with missing filaments. *Obstet. Gynecol.*, **49**, 55-60

Vessey, M. P. (1979). Risk of ectopic pregnancy and duration of use of an intrauterine device. *Lancet*, **2**, 501-2

Vessey, M. P., Doll, R., Peto, R. Johnson, B. and Wiggins, P. (1976). A long-term follow-up study of women using different methods of contraception: an interim report. *J. Biosoc. Sci.*, **8**, 373-427

Vessey, M. P., Yeates, D., Flavel, R. and McPherson, K. (1981). Pelvic inflammatory disease and the intrauterine device: findings in a large cohort study. *Br. Med. J.*, **282**, 855-7

Weekes, A. R. L. and Hutchins, C. J. (1976). Ectopic pregnancy: a 5 year review. *Br. J. Clin. Pract.*, **30,** 104-6

Westrom, L., Bengtsson, L. P. and Mardh, P. A. (1976). The risk of pelvic inflammatory disease in women using intrauterine contraceptive devices as compared to non-users. *Lancet,* **2,** 221-4

Williams, P., Johnson, B. and Vessey, M. (1975). Septic abortions in women using intra-uterine devices. *Br. Med. J.,* **4,** 263

Zakin, D., Stern, W. Z. and Rosenblatt, R. (1981). Complete and partial uterine perforation and embedding following insertion of intrauterine devices. *Obstet. Gynecol. Survey,* **36,** 401-17

Section III
TECHNICAL PROGRESS

7
Topical uterine anesthesia for IUD insertion

H. M. HASSON

INTRODUCTION

The successful use of topical anesthesia on mucous membrances in various parts of the body suggests that topical uterine anesthesia may be similarly effective. The method was previously investigated in preliminary clinical trials which confirmed its utility in alleviating discomfort caused by uterine manipulations associated with minor gynecologic procedures (Hasson, 1976).

The purpose of this report is to present additional data on the use of topical uterine anesthesia for intrauterine device (IUD) insertion.

MATERIALS AND METHODS

Two instruments were utilized to deliver the topical anesthetic solution into the uterine cavity. These were uterine cannulas formed with an acorn possessing a pliable perforated frontal tube approximately 2 mm in diameter. The initial instrument consisted of a metal adapter connected at one end with a plastic acorn and at the other end with a disposable syringe (Figure 7.1). The second and more recent instrument was a modified spring-loaded, self-holding uterine cannula with an acorn; the metal tip of the acorn was replaced by a pliable tip (Figure 7.1).

Lidocaine was the anesthetic agent used exclusively in the study. A 1% solution was employed in the first 309 applications and a 2% solution in the remaining 134 cases. 2–6 ml of the 1% solution or 2–3 ml of the 2% lidocaine solution were aspirated into a syringe through a needle. The needle was discarded and one of the topical block instruments was assembled using sterile techniques.

A bimanual examination was performed to determine uterine position and size. The cervix was held with a tenaculum and the instrument was introduced gently into the cervical canal until its acorn firmly abutted the external cervical os. The lidocaine solution was then injected slowly into the

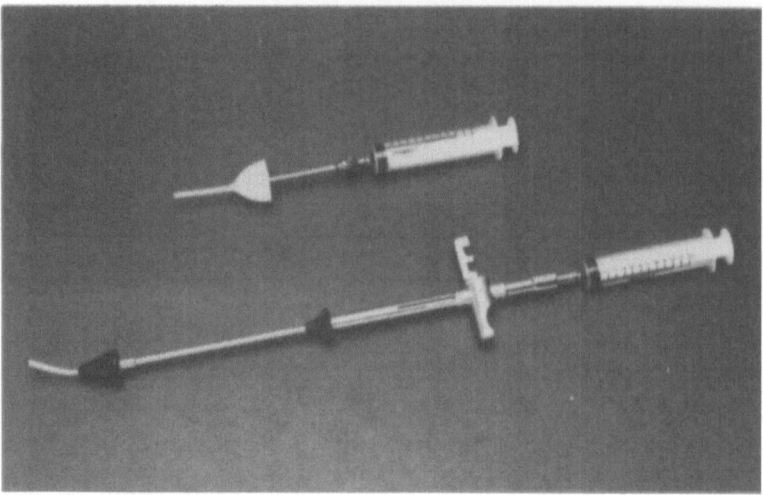

Figure 7.1 Instruments used to instill lidocaine into the uterine cavity. Hand-held model (top); self-holding device (bottom)

uterine cavity. Using the first instrument, it was necessary to hold the instrument throughout the application and to apply traction on the tenaculum with one hand while exerting pressure on the acorn with the other hand in order to prevent the escape of the anesthetic solution from the uterus and to push the acorn more deeply into the cervix. These maneuvers were not necessary with the spring-loaded, self-holding second model. In either case, the application resulted in progressive cervical dilatation as evidenced by gradual forward progression of the acorn into the cervical canal. In some multiparous women, the acorn almost disappeared into the cervix.

The acorn was maintained in position on the cervix for 2–5 min. Shorter durations of time were used in the initial phase of the study; however, it soon became apparent that duration of the application was critical to the result: optimum anesthetic effect of the lidocaine was noted at 5 min but not sooner. The 5-min duration was then employed routinely. The longer duration became more convenient with the use of the second instrument, as it was no longer necessary to hold the instrument following injection. It also became possible to leave the patient after setting a timer and return for removing the instrument at the proper time. Following removal of the instrument, uterine measurements were obtained using the Wing Sound (Hasson, 1974) and different IUDs were inserted in the usual manner.

IUD insertion could not be accomplished in four patients with cervical stenosis. The diagnosis was made early and without traumatic manipulations. When, with reasonable pressure, the 2 mm tip of either instrument did not pass through the cervical canal or internal cervical os, the diagnosis of cervical stenosis was made and the application abandoned. These cases were excluded from the study.

A history of allergy or hypersensitivity to local anesthetic agents, severe cardiac disease, epilepsy or seizures were considered contraindications. No preoperative medications were administered. Patients were asked at the end of the procedure to describe their reactions. From their responses the following categories were distinguished: procedure intolerable, operation tolerated with great discomfort, operation tolerated with moderate discomfort, procedure well tolerated with mild discomfort and procedure well tolerated without discomfort. All IUD insertions were performed by the author as intermenstrual procedures between August of 1974 and December of 1981.

RESULTS

The composition of the clinical sample is shown in Table 7.1 and the types of IUDs used in the series in Table 7.2. All patients tolerated the procedures. Satisfactory relief of pain was noted in 97.3% or 431 patients. Twelve patients or 2.7% of the sample experienced moderated discomfort and none reported great discomfort (Table 7.3).

Table 7.1 Patient characteristics (17–46 years)

Characteristic	Number	Percentage
Race		
White	371	84
Black	58	13
Oriental	14	3
Parity		
Nulliparous	248	56
Parous	195	44

Table 7.2 IUDs used in the series

Type of IUD	Number	Percentage
Cu-7	277	63
Small Cu-7	53	12
Lippes Loop	80	18
Progestasert	21	5
Dalkon Shield	8	2
Cu-T	2	0.5
Multiload	2	0.5

The study was divided into two groups: 309 patients in whom 1% lidocaine was used and 134 patients in whom 2% lidocaine was utilized (Tables 7.3, 7.4 and 7.5). When the data were analyzed, a significant difference in the expression of pain was found related to parity but not age or race. Nulliparous women complained of mild or moderate discomfort more frequently than parous women: 19.7% and 4.4% vs. 8.7% and 0.5%, respectively (Tables 7.4 and 7.5). It was also clear that the 2% lidocaine solution

Table 7.3 Degree of discomfort expressed by patients in the study

	None % No.		Mild % No.		Moderate % No.	
Group I						
($n = 309$)	79	245	18	55	3	9
Group II						
($n = 134$)	90	120	8	11	2	3
All series						
($n = 443$)	82	365	15	66	3	12

was more effective than the 1% solution even though the dose might have been the same. There was one exception: one of 60 parous women receiving the 2% solution was considered to have moderate discomfort while none of 135 parous patients receiving the 1% solution had moderate discomfort.

Table 7.4 Degree of discomfort expressed by nulliparous patients in the study

	None % No.		Mild % No.		Moderate % No.	
Group I						
($n = 174$)	71	124	24	41	5	9
Group II						
($n = 74$)	86	64	11	8	3	2
All series						
($n = 248$)	76	188	20	49	4	11

This patient had a mild vasovagal reaction during placement of a Lippes Loop D. Two other mild vasovagal reactions occurred in the series and the phenomenon was reported as moderate discomfort.

The 12 occurrences of moderate discomfort noted in the series are tabu-

Table 7.5 Degree of discomfort expressed by parous patients in the study

	None % No.		Mild % No.		Moderate % No.	
Group I						
($n = 135$)	90	121	10	14	0	
Group II						
($n = 60$)	93	56	5	3	2	1
All series						
($n = 195$)	91	177	9	17	0.5	1

lated in Table 7.6 by parity and IUD type. A surprisingly high incidence (9%) of moderate discomfort was observed in the small Copper 7 series, even though it was expected that this smaller device would be better tolerated. The explanation of this unexpected result probably relates to the

Table 7.6 12 occurrences of moderate discomfort noted in the series

Parity	Device	Observations
0	Cu-7	
0	Cu-7	
0	Cu-7	Marked apprehension observed
0	Cu-7	
0	Cu-7	Tight internal cervical os
0	Small Cu-7	Mild vasovagal reaction occurred with application of tenaculum
0	Small Cu-7	Marked apprehension noted
0	Small Cu-7	Discomfort occurred with application of tenaculum
0	Small Cu-7	
0	Small Cu-7	Mild vasovagal reaction occurred with IUD placement
0	Progestasert	
2	Loop D	Mild vasovagal reaction occurred with IUD placement

circumstances under which the insertion was carried out, as discussed later in this report.

Further study of the data indicated that, although topical uterine anesthesia was effective in reducing discomfort associated with introducing the Wing Sound or the IUD into the uterus, touching the fundus with either device, placement of the IUD in the uterine cavity and IUD postinsertion cramping, it did not affect expressions of pain related to application of the tenaculum and/or subsequent traction on the cervix. The degree of patient apprehension was alleviated only to the extent that the expectation of pain did not materialize. These observations are outlined in Table 7.7. Injection of the anesthetic solution into the uterus was associated in many patients with a mild burning or heavy sensation or mild uterine cramping that lasted for approximately 30 sec and subsided thereafter.

Table 7.7 Effect of topical uterine anesthesia on different components of discomfort associated with IUD insertion

Potential pain component	Relieved by topical uterine anesthesia	Not relieved by topical uterine anesthesia
(1) Application of tenaculum on cervix		+
(2) Traction on cervix		+
(3) Passage of sound or device through internal cervical os	+	
(4) Touching the fundus with sound or device	+	
(5) Placement of IUD	+	
(6) Uterine distentions by IUD	±	
(7) Postinsertion discomfort	+	
(8) Apprehension		+*

*Apprehension may be reduced when the expectation of pain does not materialize

Complications

No complications or adverse reactions attributable to the topical anesthetic were noted in the series. The three instances of mild vasovagal reactions were attributed to the degree of patient apprehension and/or failure of the method to alleviate discomfort.

DISCUSSION

Topical anesthesia is utilized with considerable success on the mucous membrane of the oropharynx, conjunctiva, respiratory and urinary tracts and the anus. However, the use of this anesthetic modality in the field of gynecology has remained largely unexplored.

In 1975, Munsick reported a well conducted double blind study in which he applied the anesthetic agent tetracaine in a 1% solution on the cervix and instilled the solution into the uterine cavity prior to IUD insertion. Munsick concluded that tetracaine had no topical anesthetic effect on the cervix or uterus. It would appear, however, that the choice of anesthetic agent and method of its application determined the outcome. Effective topical anesthesia could not have been accomplished with the methods reported by Munsick, for the following reasons:

(1) Whereas the efficacy of local anesthetics on mucous membranes has been established, their effect on epithelial barriers has not. Therefore, in nine of 17 paired applications where only response to tenaculum placement on the cervix was studied, no anesthetic effect could have been expected.

(2) In the remaining applications, the anesthetic solution was instilled into the uterine cavity but it was permitted to leak out through the cervix, since no mechanism was provided to retain the solution within the cavity following injection. Furthermore, the procedures of cervical dilation and IUD insertion were initiated 2 min after the injection. Since the anesthetic effect of tetracaine requires an average latency period of 9 min (compared to 4 min for lidocaine) and adequate tissue contact to permit absorption by the mucous membrane, and since these prerequisites were not met in the Munsick study, adequate anesthetic effect could not have been anticipated.

Following my initial study, the technique of topical uterine anesthesia was used successfully by other investigators (Schellen, 1983; van Santen and Haspels, 1981).

Satisfactory relief of pain associated with IUD insertion was reported by 97% of all patients enrolled in this study. As expected, parous women voiced fewer complaints than nulliparous. Only one of 195 parous women or 0.5% had moderate discomfort as compared to 11 of 248 nulliparous women or 4%. When the data were analyzed by IUD type, it was surprising to find that insertion of the small Cu-7 was associated with an exceptionally high rate (9%) of moderate discomfort. This finding is probably related to greater patient apprehension rather than to any inherent features of the device at the time of insertion. The small Copper 7 was an investigational device and many patients, despite attempts to allay their fears, were concerned with using an 'experimental' IUD.

94

Topical uterine anesthesia is not expected to significantly alter expressions of pain attributed to patient apprehension. Reassurance and/or the administration of a tranquillizer or a sedative would be more appropriate. Although painful sensations associated with application of a tenaculum on the cervix are not common and the subject of sensitivity of the ectocervix is debatable, any such sensations are not expected to be alleviated with topical use of lidocaine since this agent does not appear to penetrate epithelial barriers.

The reported technique produced a reasonable amount of cervical dilatation. This benefit was not anticipated. Initially, it was thought that cervical dilatation was predominantly caused by mechanical wedging of the acorn into the cervix. Subsequently I performed several hysterosalpingograms using the same instrument and technique but without instilling lidocaine solution into the uterine cavity. I did not observe any appreciable degree of cervical dilation under such conditions. Thus, it is tempting to surmise that the injected lidocaine was absorbed through the mucous membrane of the endocervix and caused a relaxing effect on the 'cervical sphincter'. Making an early diagnosis of cervical stenosis without traumatic manipulations is considered to be another advantage of the reported instrument and method.

Lack of a practical objective method for evaluating anesthetic activity of topically applied local anesthetics is a problem (Adriani and Zepernick, 1964). A comparative double-blind study is also needed to verify our results. Following my preliminary report, a multicenter double-blind study sponsored by a leading manufacturer of lidocaine was planned. Unfortunately, requirements of regulatory agencies dissuaded the sponsor from conducting the study. However, during the past 7 years I have performed, for one reason or another, some 40 IUD fittings using the Wing Sound and various IUDs without topical anesthesia. Many of the patients, particularly nulliparous patients, did not tolerate the procedures well. Berger et al. (1976) inserted Lippes Loop A or B, Dalkon Shield or Copper 7 IUDs in 93 nulliparous patients without anesthesia of any type. They reported a 42.5% incidence of cramping during IUD insertion and 34.4% rate of moderate or severe pain immediately after the insertion. The value of topical uterine anesthesia can be appreciated when these results are compared to those of the present study.

The absence of complications in this series is reassuring. However, the methods described here must be followed closely to ensure safety. The use of other local anesthetic agents, doses or techniques may not prove satisfactory. The topical use of local anesthetic agents represents an extremely complex subject. Anesthetic activity varies as a function of the agent, the form and concentration of application and the site of administration. Certain local anesthetics are relatively potent when injected, but rather weak when applied topically and vice versa. Potential toxicity also varies considerably by type of agent, dose, type and vascularity of mucous membranes and surface area of the topical application. For instance, the rate of absorption of tetracaine from mucous membranes approaches that of intravenous administration and numerous fatalities have resulted from its topical use for endoscopic procedures (Adriani and Campbell, 1956). The cause of death was frequently attributed to over-dosage from rapid absorption.

Lidocaine is a member of the amide group of local anesthetics. It does not appear to penetrate epithelial barriers but is readily absorbed from mucous membranes. The local anesthetic activity of lidocaine appears to be comparable when the agent is used for local infiltration or topical application; however, the rate of systemic absorption from mucous membranes is more rapid. When applied topically, lidocaine has a general latency period of 3–5 min and a duration of action of 30–60 min. The drug is hydrolyzed in the liver and its metabolites are excreted by the kidney (Covino, 1972a, b).

In this study, the dose of lidocaine used for topical uterine anesthesia was limited to 60 mg. The maximum dose for topical application in other sites was reported to be 200 mg. While increasing the dose may enhance the anesthetic effect in topical uterine applications, it may also bring about undesirable side-effects.

The toxic reactions of lidocaine are manifested through its cardiovascular and central nervous system actions. With increasing blood levels, myocardial contractility and cardiac output decrease while peripheral vasodilatation increases. These combined effects result in systemic hypotension. Toxic levels of lidocaine depress cardiac conduction leading ultimately to cardiac arrest. Increasing blood levels of lidocaine also cause central nervous system excitation manifested clinically as tremors, shivering and ultimately convulsions. A further elevation of blood drug levels results in generalized central nervous system depression and, finally, respiratory arrest (Covino, 1972a).

Although occasional cases of suspected allergy have been reported, true allergic reactions to local anesthetic agents, particularly those of the amide type, are extremely rare (Aldrete and Johnson, 1964; Covino, 1972a). It should be noted that use of excessive dosage or epinephrine can lead to reactions that may not be easily distinguished from those associated with systemic anaphylaxis. The use of epinephrine in topical uterine applications should be strictly avoided.

CONCLUSIONS

When used as described, topical uterine anesthesia is safe and effective in minimizing pain associated with IUD insertion. The instrument and method have the additional advantage of causing a reasonable amount of cervical dilatation and of making an early atraumatic diagnosis of cervical stenosis.

References

Adriani, J. and Campbell, D. (1956). Fatalities following topical applications of local anesthetics to mucous membranes. *J. Am. Med. Assoc.*, **162**, 1527–30
Adriani, J. and Zepernick, R. (1964). Clinical effectiveness of drugs used for topical anesthesia. *J. Am. Med. Assoc.*, **188**, 711–16

Aldrete, J.A. and Johnson, D.A. (1970). Evaluation of intracutaneous testing for investigation of allergy to local anesthetic agents. *Anesth. Analg.*, **49**, 173–83

Berger, G.S., Edelman, D.A. and Reginie, S.J. (1976). Patients' responses to IUD insertion. *Int. J. Gynaecol. Obstet.*, **14**, 147–9

Covino, B.G. (1972a). Local anesthesia (I). *N. Eng. J. Med.*, **286**, 975–83

Covino, B.G. (1972b). Local anesthesia (II). *N. Engl. J. Med.*, **286**, 1035–42

Hasson, H.M. (1974). Clinical applications of the Wing Sound device. *Obstet. Gynecol.*, **43**, 498–506

Hasson, H.M. (1976). Topical uterine anesthesis. A preliminary report. *Int. J. Gynaecol. Obstet.*, **15**, 238–40

Munsick, R.A. (1975). Topical anesthesia of the uterine cervix or corpus. *Obstet. Gynecol.* **46**, 613–15

van Santen, M.R. and Haspels, A.A. (1981). Interception by post-coital IUD insertion. *Contracept. Deliv. Syst.*, **2**, 189–200

Schellen, T.C.M. (1983) Intrauterine anesthesia: a new approach. *Int. J. Fertil.*, **28**, 57–8

8
Ultrasonography for predicting correct location of the IUD

G. BERNASCHEK and R. SPERNOL

The intrauterine device (IUD) represents a highly reliable method of contraception, provided that the device is properly placed in the uterine cavity. Ultrasonography (USG) is a new technology that is capable of improving IUD performance by investigating anatomic characteristics of the uterine cavity prior to IUD insertion and by identifying the position of the device within the cavity following insertion. With USG it is also possible to distinguish the type of IUD used, if the information is not available. For example, the Copper T displays a strong echo, representing the vertical arm on longitudinal sonographic section within the uterine cavity (Figure 8.1). Such a typical echo can be found in patients with Copper 7 and Nova T. Depending on the resolution quality of the scanner, even the loops of the copper wire can sometimes be indentified. Transverse sections show the horizontal arms of these models (Figures 8.2, 8.3, 8.4). Lippes Loops are identified by their characteristic interrupted echoes indicating their spiral shape (Figure 8.5).

STUDIES ON NON-PREGNANT IUD CARRIERS

We have examined 169 non-pregnant women wearing IUDs in order to identify the position of the device within the uterine cavity and to establish criteria for correct fitting based on the distance between the upper end of the device and the uterine fundus. In each patient, the following parameters were studied: uterine length, uterine position, thickness of anterior and posterior walls and the distance between the upper end of the IUD and the fundus. The data were subsequently evaluated for statistical significance.

The clinical sample consisted of 31 nulliparous women (18.3%), 56 uniparous (33.1%) and 82 (48.6%) multiparous women. The uterus was anteverted in 154 patients (91.1%), anteversion was associated with marked anteflexion in 33 patients. Uterine retroversion was noted in the remaining 15 women; this was associated with additional retroflexion in 14 of the 15 women. The total length of the uterus varied from 60 mm to 133 mm, the

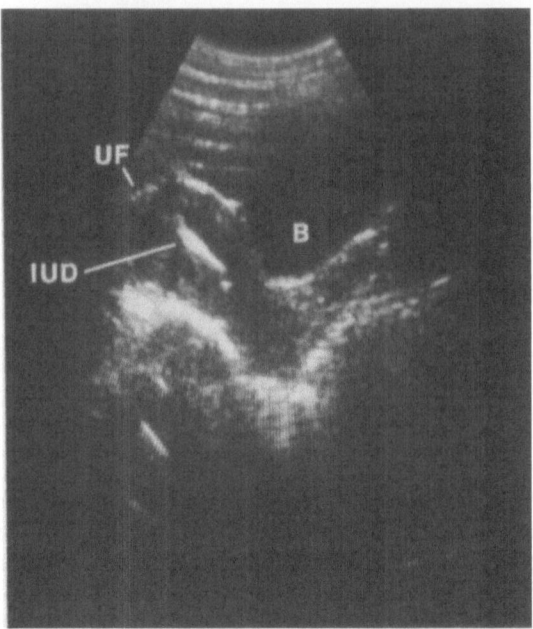

Figure 8.1. Longitudinal section demonstrating the vertical arm of the IUD (B = bladder; UF = uterine fundus)

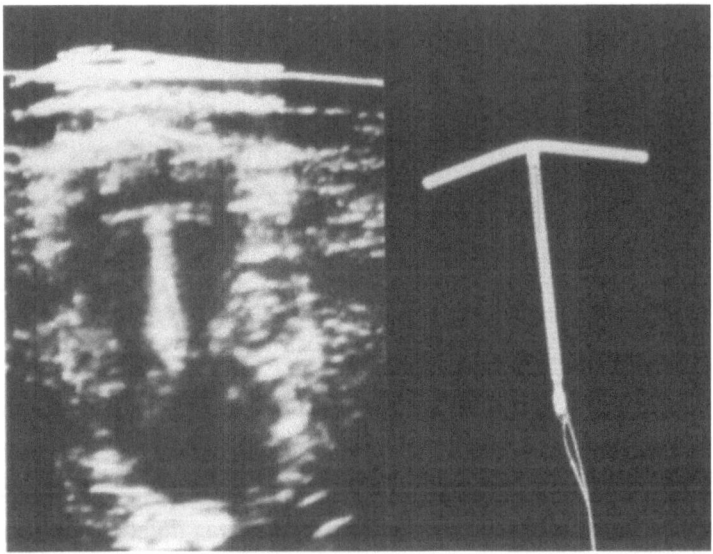

Figure 8.2 Transverse section demonstrating a Copper T *in situ*

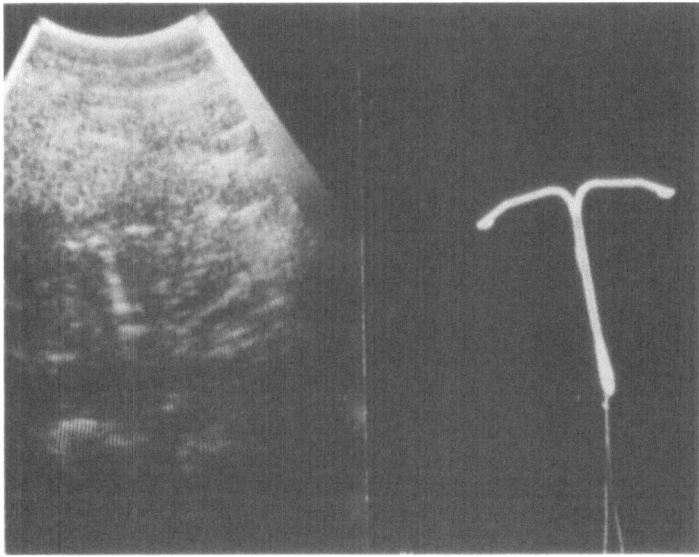

Figure 8.3 Transverse section showing a Nova T *in situ*

mean was 83 mm. The difference between the mean length in nulliparous women (76.2 mm) and in women having delivered once (80.5 mm) was significant ($p = 0.009$). There was also a highly significant difference ($p = 0.0001$) between the mean length of the uterus in uniparous and multiparous women (87.4) mm).

To establish the optimal distance between the uterine fundus and the

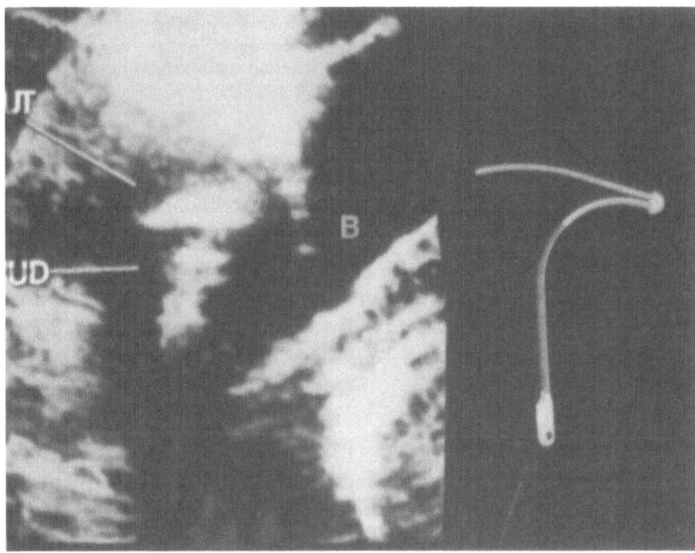

Figure 8.4 Transverse section showing a Copper 7 *in situ*

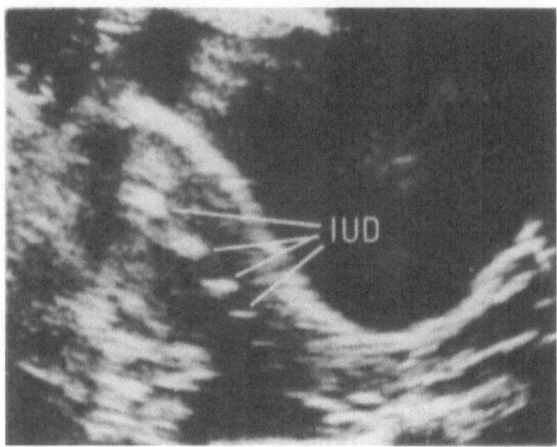

Figure 8.5   Longitudinal scan in a case with Lippes Loop

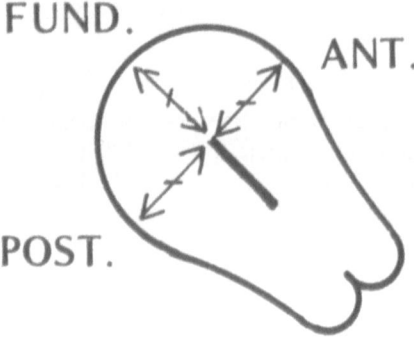

Figure 8.6   Various distances measured on a longitudinal section prove correct location of an IUD

upper end of the IUD, we have considered individual variations in the thickness of the uterine wall, an element that has been previously neglected. We compared the thickness of the anterior and posterior wall of the uterus, as determined on longitudinal sonographic sections (Figure 8.6). According to our calculations, the IUD is considered to be correctly located if the distance between its upper end and the uterine fundus is not greater than the thickness of the uterine wall plus one-third. Figure 8.7 shows that the distribution curves of the three measured values are almost equal. In patients with a great distance between the IUD and the fundus, for example, women with the IUD in the cervix (Figure 8.8), the incorrect position can be diagnosed by the distribution diagram. Detection of improperly placed IUDs with their upper end in the center of the uterine cavity (Figure 8.9) is also possible by means of these curves. If we correlate the distance between the IUD and the fundus with the thickness of the anterior and posterior uterine wall we find a far-reaching conformity of these three

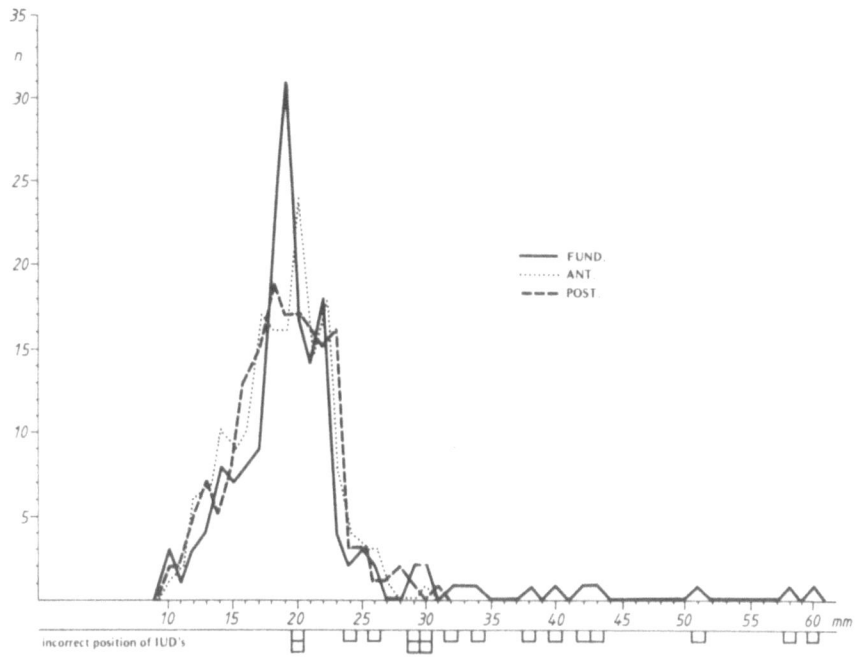

Figure 8.7 Distribution curves of the thickness of the anterior (ANT) and the posterior (POST) uterine wall and the distance between the upper end of the IUD from the fundus uteri (FUND) uterine wall and the distance between the upper end of the IUD from the fundus uteri (FUND)

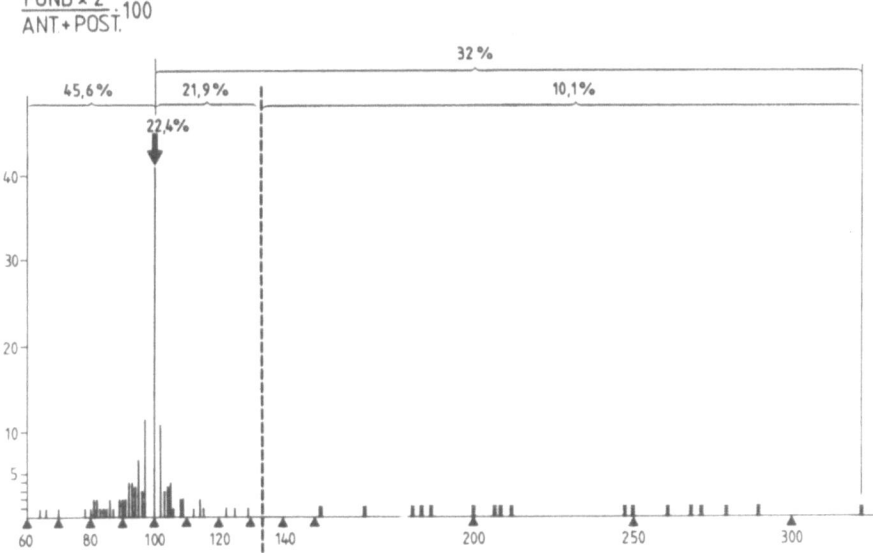

Figure 8.8 Correlation between the distance from the fundus uteri and the anterior and posterior uterine wall thickness

103

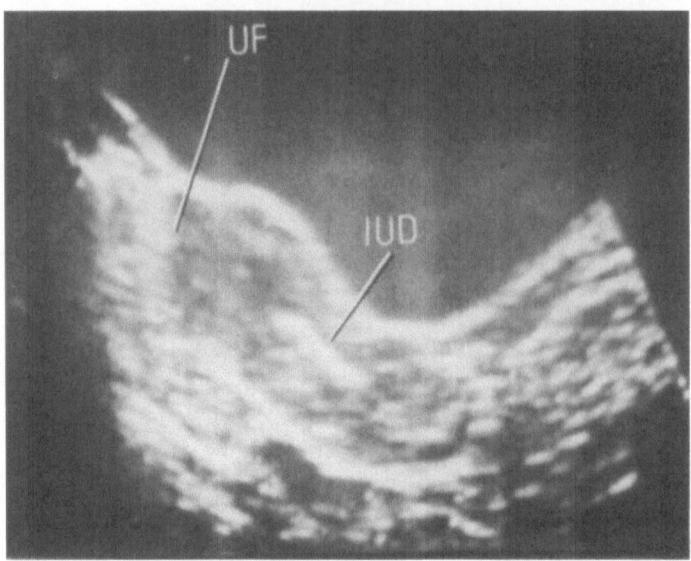

Figure 8.9 Longitudinal scan showing an IUD with the upper end in the center of the uterine cavity. The distance from the fundus uteri (UF) exceeds the thickness of the uterine wall by more than one-third

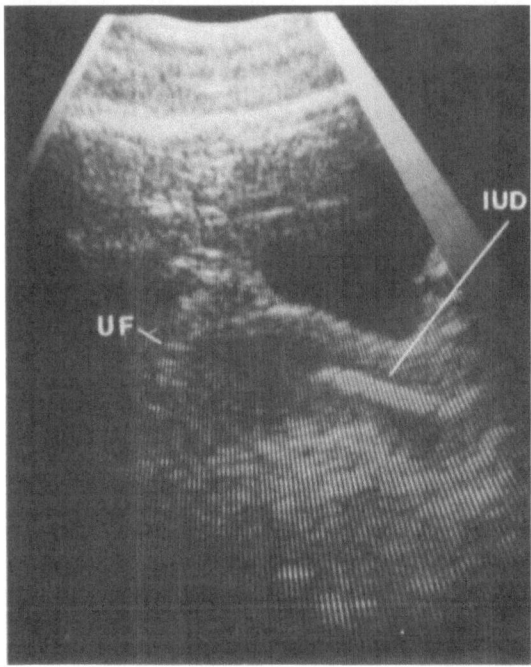

Figure 8.10 IUD lying in the cervical canal (UF = uterine fundus)

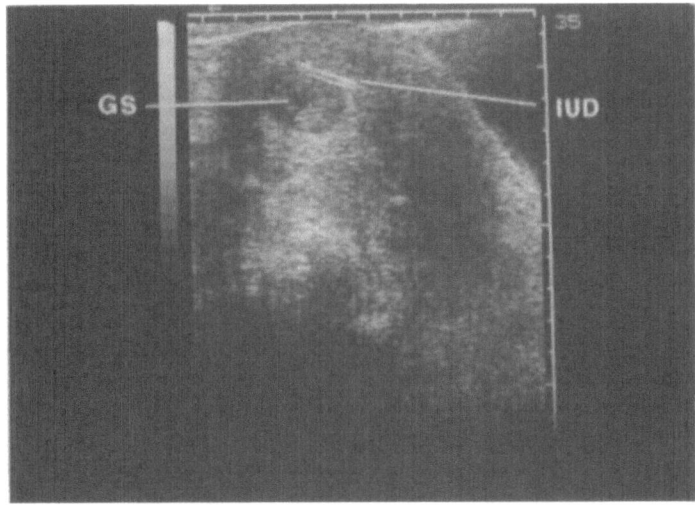

Figure 8.11 Pregnancy despite correctly located IUD (GS = gestational sac)

parameters in a vast majority of the cases. A marked flattening of the distribution curve is observed only when the distance between the fundus and the IUD exceeds the thickness of the anterior or posterior uterine wall by more than one-third (Figure 8.10). Using the above-mentioned criteria, 17 women with improperly placed IUDs were identified among the 169 patients examined. The distance from the fundus uteri varied between 20 mm and 60 mm. In women showing incorrect location of the IUD, the

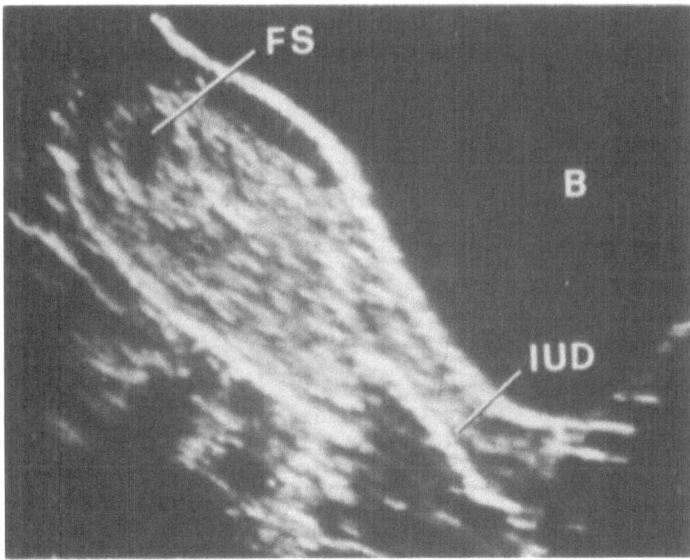

Figure 8.12 Longitudinal scan in a pregnant woman; the IUD is lying in the cervical canal (GS = gestational sac; B = bladder)

uterine length was significantly shorter ($p = 0.01$), irrespective of parity; in some multiparous women the length of the uterus was below the average.

STUDIES ON IUD PATIENTS WITH A MISSING TAIL OR PREGNANCY

Disappearance of the IUD tail or control thread may be due to pregnancy. The importance of improper IUD position in increasing the risk of pregnancy was demonstrated by our previous work (Bernaschek et al., 1981). The IUD was found to be located correctly within the uterine cavity in only 11 of 59 women who became pregnant while using the device (Figure 8.11). In 40 patients who were less than 9 weeks pregnant, the IUD was located in the cervical canal or in the lower third of the uterus (Figure 8.12). Eight women whose pregnancies were greater than 9 weeks gestation were excluded because of possible secondary displacement of the pessary as a consequence of the enlarging uterus and gestational sac. These findings indicate that the contraceptive effect of IUDs is strongly dependent upon the position of the device within the uterine cavity. The distance between the upper end of the device and the uterine fundus, as measured by ultrasound, may be utilized to predict the degree of safety concerning contraceptive efficacy of the IUD (Meyenburg, 1978; Schmidt et al., 1979).

Many clinicians estimate uterine position of the IUD by observing the length of its tail within the vagina. This method is not adequate: a developing pregnancy may cause the IUD to rise into the uterine cavity if the enlarging gestational sac is situated either below or lateral to the device, or it may displace the device into the cervical canal if the implantation site is above the IUD.

In women with a missing thread the IUD need not be removed if the ultrasound examination shows a correct intrauterine location of the IUD. Nevertheless, this method of follow-up requires frequent sonographic examinations (Wahren and Schlensker, 1980). A diagnosis of perforation can be made only if the IUD is seen partly in the uterus. An empty uterus alone should not lead to the assumption that the IUD has been expelled; X-ray examination is obligatory to identify a possibly symptomless extra-uterine IUD that might be located between loops of bowel, where it cannot be detected by ultrasound.

CONCLUSION

On the basis of our studies we recommend the following applications for USG in association with IUD use:

(1) A sonographic exploration of the uterine anatomy before insertion of the IUD to exclude women whose uterus is too small and to help in selecting appropriate IUD size.

(2) A control USG examination immediately after IUD insertion to detect incorrect location early.

(3) Check-ups after 3 or 6 months, because dislocation and expulsion are observed mostly during the first few months after insertion.

(4) A control USG examination in women complaining of pain or amenorrhea, to locate the IUD relative to a possible gestational sac and to detect dislocation of the IUD.

REFERENCES

Bernaschek, G., Spernol, R. and Beck, A. (1981). IUD-Lage bei intrauterinene Schwangerschaften. *Geburtsh. Frauenheilk.*, **41,** 645-7

Meyenburg, H (1978). Anwendung der Ultraschall-Schnittbildtechnik zur Darstellung von Intrauterinpessaren. *Geburtsh. Frauenheilk.*, **38,** 950

Schmidt, E. H., Wagner, H., Quakernack, K. and Beller, F. K. (1979). Ergebnisse der Lageüberwachung von Intrauterinpessaren durch Ultraschall. *Geburtsh. Frauenheilk.* **39,** 138-43

Wahren, J. and Schlensker, K. H. (1980). Ultraschalldiagnostik bei Komplikationen durch Intrauterinspiralen. Presented at the *43rd Meeting of the Deutschen Gesellschaft für Gynäkolologie und Geburtshilfe,* Hamburg

9
Ultrasonography for preventing accidental pregnancy due to IUD displacement

S. LEVI

Ultrasonography of the female pelvis shows the contours and structure of the genital organs, including cervix and corpus uteri, myometrium and cavity. Diagnostic ultrasound is non-invasive and harmless—important advantages in the woman with an unsuspected pregnancy. With ultrasonography (USG), the presence of an intrauterine contraceptive device (IUD) in the uterus can be assessed and its position demonstrated (Cochrane and Thomas, 1972; Ianniruberto and Mastrobernardino, 1972; Janssens et al., 1973; Nemes and Kerenyi, 1971; Piiroinen, 1972; Winters, 1966). IUD misplacement, displacement or loss is probably a frequent cause of unintentional pregnancies. Visualization of IUD strings gives information only on the presence of the IUD, not on its position. If the string is not visible, the IUD may have been expelled or may have perforated the uterine wall. The retraction of the string is not uncommon. Ultrasonic visualization and location of the IUD at regular intervals should help to avoid accidental pregnancies in unprotected or less protected women. We therefore asked colleagues in our clinic to send patients wearing an IUD for an ultrasonic check-up. The results of our observations of such patients during 26 months are reported here.

MATERIALS AND METHODS

A continuous series of 750 patients wearing an IUD had regular ultrasound evaluations to determine the precise position of the device. The USG examination was occasionally performed for suspected pelvic abnormality such as pain, hemorrhage, swelling, abnormal menstruation or bleeding, or suspected pregnancy. Patient age ranged from 19 to 50 years, gestity varied between 0 and 10 and parity between 0 and 8. In our lab, we prefer to use the sector scan for pelvic check-up because it gives a good view of the pelvic area and allows a very quick procedure (mechanical real time sector scan 2.5 MHz Combison 100 Kretz). The examination is eventually continued with another scanner, if a pregnancy or large tumor is to be examined

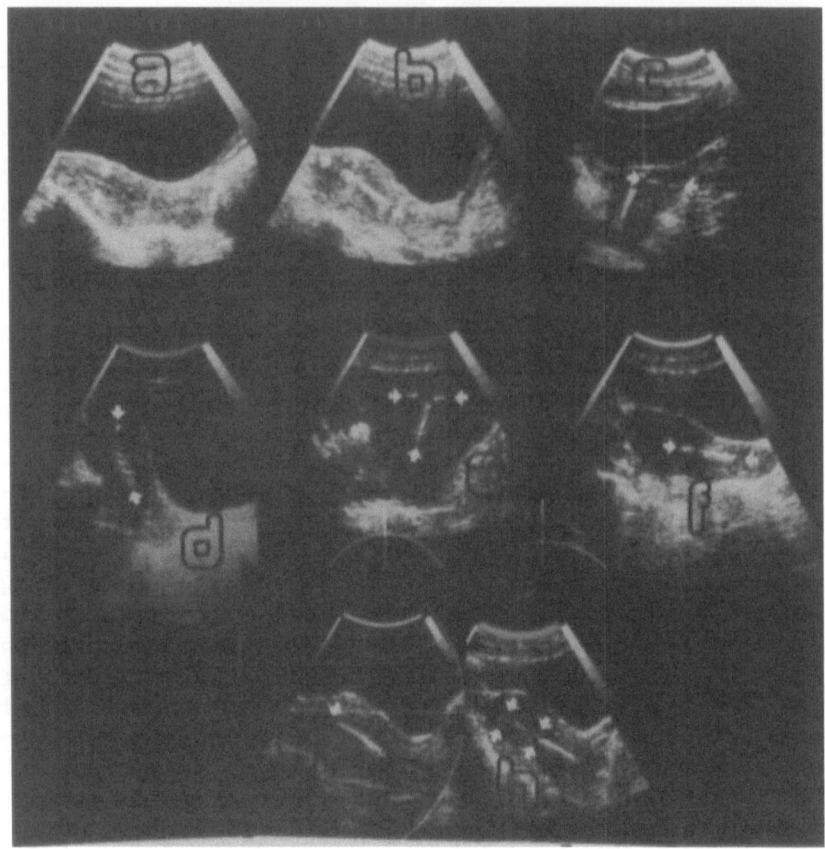

Figure 9.1 Longitudinal scans of uterus. (a) Usual display of uterus showing surface, muscular and mucosal layers, cavity (virtual) between white arrows; (b),(g) IUD normally located in uterine cavity (between arrows); (c) IUD in retroverted uterus (string is visible, arrow); (d) five dots of Lippes Loop (between arrows); (e) cephalad sections of uterus, head, body of IUD between arrows; (f),(h) low-lying IUD. Arrows underline empty part of uterine cavity

(electronic real time linear array 3.5 MHz Superscan 50 Kontron and UI Octoson Ausonics). Longitudinal and transverse sections are routinely performed while the patient has a full bladder. Uterine position, size and contours, as well as the tissue layers and cavity, are part of the routine examination (Figure 9.1a). IUDs are displayed in longitudinal section as a straight line of intense echoes (Figure 9.1b). A Lippes Loop device is displayed by five dots (Figure 9.1d). On transverse scans, the IUD reflects sound as a bright point (Figure 9.2a). The transverse cephalad oblique section shows the specific shape of the inserted IUD (Figure 9.1e, Figure 9.3). This is particularly true for T- and 7-shaped IUDs and much less for more flexible heads, such as the Multiload. A cephalad scan of the uterus is not always obtainable.

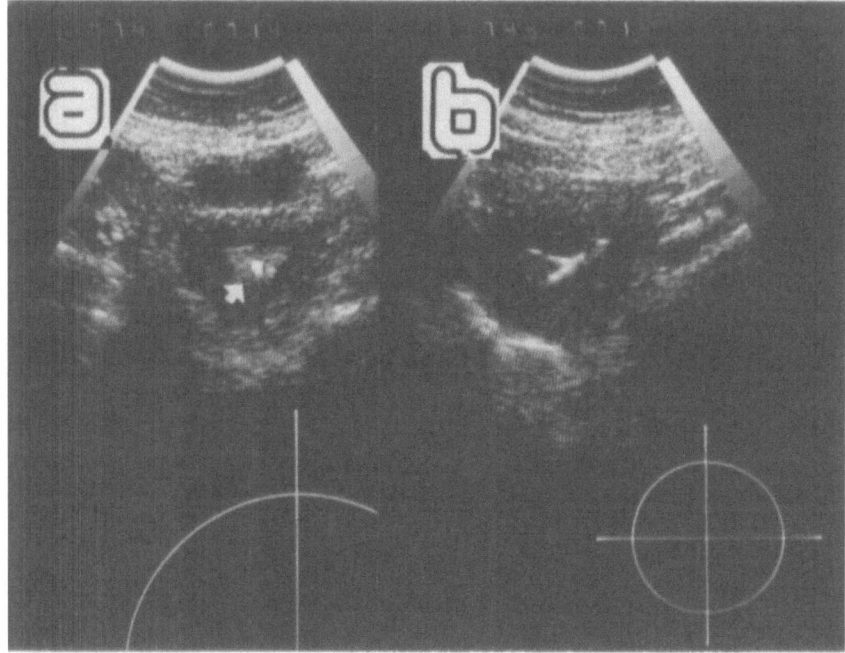

Figure 9.2 Transverse scans of uterus. (a) IUD is bright dot at centre of uterus surrounded by echoes of relatively high amplitude (possibly due to endometritis); (b) displaced IUD in oblique position

The position of the IUD in the cavity is ordinarily shown by longitudinal sections only, but may be confirmed, if necessary, by scans performed in other planes.

The IUD is assumed to occupy its normal location when the echoes are high within the cavity, the distance between the bottom of the cavity and the IUD not exceeding 5-7 mm (Figures 9.1b-e and 9.3). The IUD is diag-

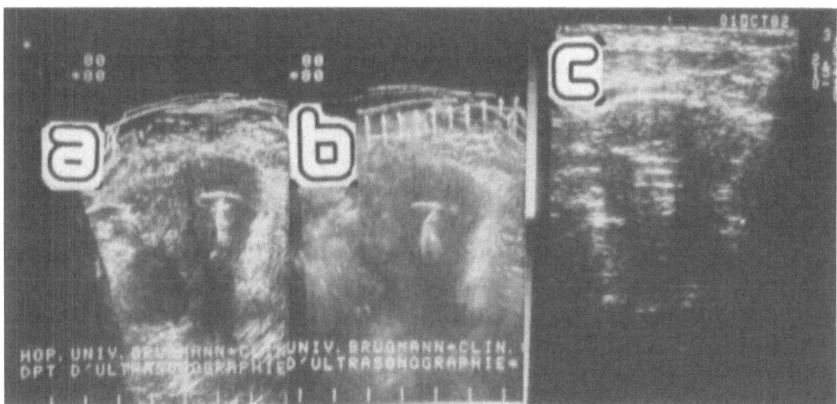

Figure 9.3 Cephalid transverse scans. (a) T-shaped IUD; (b) 7-shaped IUD; (c) Lippes Loop

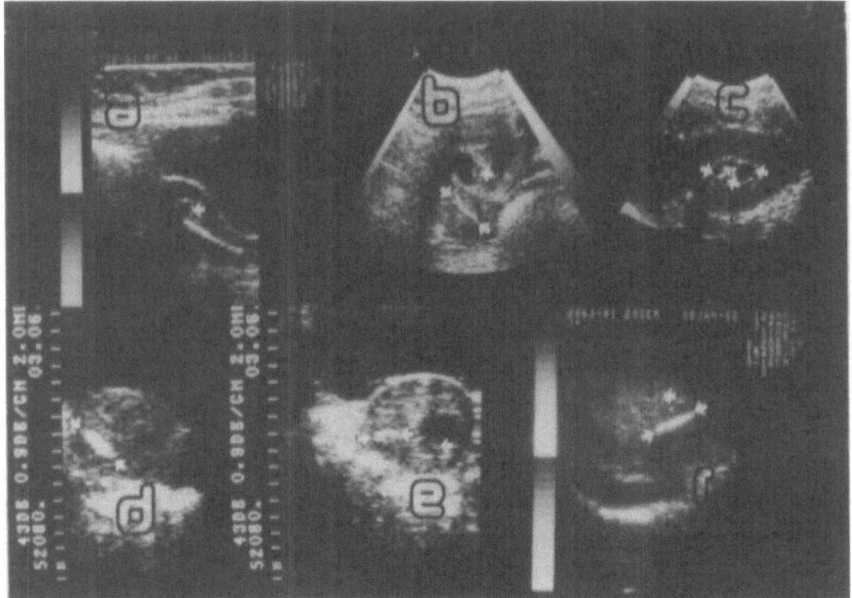

Figure 9.4 IUD in pregnant women. (a) 5-Week pregnancy (arrow) with IUD 5 mm away from fundus; (b) 6-week pregnancy and embryo (arrow) with cervical IUD (arrows); (c) 4-week pregnancy and pseudogestation sac (arrows), IUD in cavity (arrows) in woman with ectopic pregnancy; (d),(e) laterally-pushed IUD and 6-week pregnancy; (f) IUD (arrows) lying on placenta (arrows) in 20-week pregnancy

nosed as being in the isthmic portion when the lowest 10 mm of the IUD body are at least in the cervical canal (Figures 9.1f, h and 9.4a, b). A missing IUD is not visible on the uterine scans. Some artifacts may occur. High amplitude echoes may mimic IUDs. These result from gas, air or contrast liquid during X-ray hysterograms, endometrial biopsy or curettage.

RESULTS

Selected characteristics of the population sample are shown in Tables 9.1 and 9.2. The majority of women in our sample (72%) had not undergone abortion before choosing the IUD for contraception, 22% reported one abortion, 3% two abortions and fewer than 3% had 3 or more abortions. Time between IUD placement and ultrasound examination ranged from 1 week to 15 years, mean time was around 8 months (Table 9.3).

Five IUDs were most commonly seen in our study, Gyne T (24%), Multiload (23%), Nova T (13%), Gravigard (8%) and Lippes Loop (2%). Other and unknown models were grouped together (31%) (Table 9.4, Figure 9.5).

The IUD was visible and localized in 745 of the 759 women (98%), 693 were located in the uterine cavity (91%), 53 were low, at the cervical–isthmic level (7%). In 13 women, the IUD was not visible (2%) (Table 9.5). Only one IUD was shown by X-ray to be in the abdominal cavity; it had been

Table 9.1 Age distribution of the sample

Age	n	%
1. ≥ 19	10	1.3
2. 20–24	102	15.0
3. 25–29	190	25.4
4. 30–34	196	26.2
5. 35–39	132	17.6
6. 40–44	64	8.6
7. ≤ 45	44	5.9

localized in the low isthmic position 1 week before, and thereafter was not visible.

In one woman, mid-uterine echoes stronger than normal were reflected by the cavity but these echoes were weaker than those usually reflected by an IUD. The IUD was located in the cavity; the cause of the weak reflection was not elucidated. In one woman, two IUDs were in the uterine cavity. In two women, the IUDs were in a transverse rather than a longitudinal position (Figure 9.2b). Seven of 693 patients with a corporeally located IUD had an intrauterine pregnancy, and one showed an ectopic pregnancy (Figure 9.4c–e).

Of 53 patients in whom the IUD was low, 11 were pregnant, one with an ectopic pregnancy (Figure 9.4c). Among 13 women where no IUD was visible, three were pregnant (Tables 9.6, 9.7).

Considering the whole sample, 9% of the patients had a mislocation or missing IUD, and these women had 64% of the accidental pregnancies, unaware that they were not adequately protected against pregnancy.

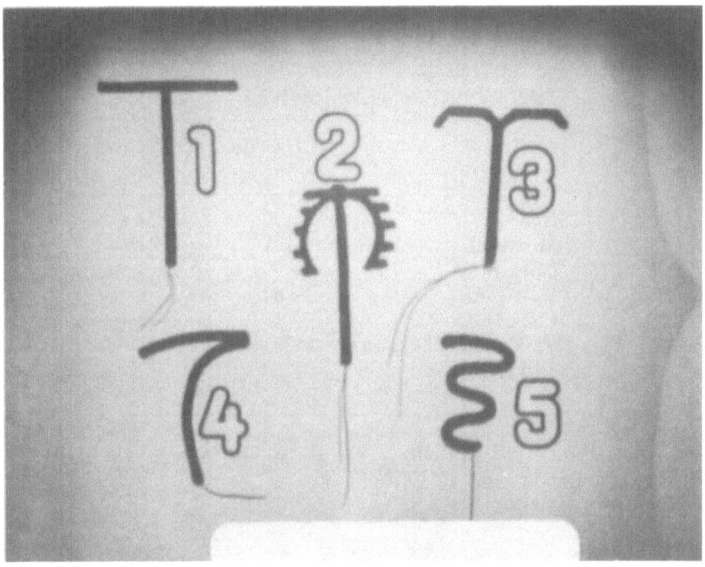

Figure 9.5 Major IUDs in study. (1) Gyne T; (2) Multiload Cu 250; (3) Nova T; (4) Gravigard; (5) Lippes Loop

Table 9.2 Difference between gravidity and parity in the sample

$P=G=n$ $n=544$		$nP=(n+1)G$ $n=165$		$nP=(n+m)G$ $n=45$	
n	%	n	%	n	%
0	23	0	16	0	. 10
1	31	1	26	1	29
2	33	2	42	2	43
3	8	3	10	3	14
4+	5	4+	6	4+	5
					$m \geq 2$

Table 9.3 Time between IUD placement and USG examination

Months	No. of cases	%
−1	182	34.3
2	67	12.7
3	44	8.4
4	19	3.7
5	16	3.0
6	21	4.0
1-11	59	11.1
12-24	98	18.4
25-36	17	3.1
37+	7	1.4
	530	100.0

Table 9.4 IUD models in the study

	IUD model n	Distribution (%)
Gyne T	179	24
Multiload	171	23
Nova T	95	13
Gravigard	64	8
Lippes Loop	15	2
Various and unknown	235	31
	759	101

Tables 9.8 and 9.9 show the time between IUD placement and USG examination by model and IUD location.

COMMENTS

Because of significant improvements in ultrasonic image qualities since the first studies of IUD location were published, the reliability of IUD detection

Table 9.5 IUD location and accidental pregnancies

	No pregnancy	Pregnancy	Total (%)
In the cavity	685(99%)	8(1%)	693(100%)
	93%	36%	91%
Cervico-isthmic location	42(79%)	11(21%)	53(100%)
	6%	50%	7%
IUD not visualized	10(77%)	3(23%)	13(100%)
	1%	14%	2%
Total	737(97%)	22(3%)	759(100%)
%	100%	100%	100%

Table 9.6 Relation between IUD location and the occurence of pregnancy

IUD location and occurrences of pregnancy	ML 250	Gyn T	Grav 7	Nova T	LL	Various/ unknown	Total
Cavity	155	154	53	89	13	229	693
No pregnancy	152	151	53	89	13	227	685
Pregnancy	3	3	0	0	0	2	8
Isthmus	14	19	10	5	1	4	53
No pregnancy	12	16	7	4	1	2	42
Pregnancy	2	3	3	1	0	2	11
Missing	2	6	1	1	1	2	13
No Pregnancy	2	5	1	0	1	1	10
Pregnancy	0	1	0	1	0	1	3
Total	171	179	64	95	15	235	759
No pregnancy	166	172	61	93	15	230	737
Pregnancy	5	7	3	2	0	5	22

with USG is no longer questionable. Currently, the presence of a device in the uterine cavity can be clearly demonstrated. The only case where precise IUD location may be difficult is the retroverted uterus (Figure 9.1c). Perforation of the uterine wall can be visualized, unless the IUD lies free in the abdominal cavity, where it can be ultrasonically detected only by chance.

The relationship between IUD position within the uterine cavity and contraceptive efficacy is shown in Table 9.5. Of 693 women with an IUD in normal position, only 1% became pregnant whereas 21% and 23% of the women with low-lying or missing IUDs, respectively, became pregnant. This is highly significant. The difference of average durations between IUD placement and USG was not significant (8.2 months for IUD in cavity, 8.9 and 8.8 months for low and missing IUDs).

The Pearl Index for pregnancy for the different groups was 1.8 when the IUD was located in the corporeal cavity, 26.4 when the IUD was in the cervical - isthmic portion, and 67.9 when the device was missing. These values support the relation of accidental pregnancy to IUD mislocation (Table 9.10).

We believe, therefore, that an USG check-up may be useful in locating an IUD with the first procedure performed 1 or 2 months after insertion,

Table 9.7   Contraception with IUD complicated by pregnancies

Case no.	Time between IUD insertion and USC exam. (months)	Model	Location
1	2	Grav 7	Isthmic
2	2	ML Cu 250	Corpus (ectop.pregn)
3	3	Gyne T	Isthmic
4	5	Grav. 7	Isthmic
5	5	ML Cu 250	Corpus
6	6	ML Cu 250	Corpus
7	8	Nova T	Isthmic
8	12	?	Missing
9	12	Gyne T	Corpus
10	14	Nova T	Missing
11	15	ML Cu 250	Isthmic
12	16	Gyne T	Corpus
13	15	Gyne T	Isthmic
14	18	Gyne T	Missing
15	24	ML Cu 250	Isthmic
16	36	Gyne T	Corpus
17	?	Grav 7	Isthmic
18	?	Gyne T	Isthmic (ectop.pregn)
19	?	?	Corpus
20	?	?	Corpus
21	?	?	Isthmic
22	?	?	Isthmic

Table 9.8   Time between IUD placement and USG examination (in months)

	n	Total	Mean
Cavity	478	3937	8.2
Isthmus	46	409	8.9
Missing	6	53	8.8
	530	4399	8.3

and subsequently, at 1-year intervals. Abnormalities, such as ovarian cysts or leiomyomata, could also be identified at the time of IUD location. The USG could thus help to reduce the number of accidental pregnancies, an avoidable complication when intrauterine devices are used for contraception.

References

Cochrane, W. D. and Thomas, M. A. (1972). The use of ultrasound B-mode scanning in the localization of intrauterine contraceptive devices. *Radiology*, **104,** 623–7

Ianniruberto, A. and Mastrobernardino, A (1972). Ultrasonic localization of the Lippes Loop. *Am. J. Obstet. Gynecol.*, **114,** 78–82

Janssens, D., Vrijens, M., Thiery, M. and Van Kets, H. (1973). Ultrasonic detection, localization and identification of intrauterine contraceptive devices. *Contraception*, **8,** 485–95

Table 9.9 Time between IUD placement and USG examination (months) by device

Model	Location	No. of patients	Mean	SD	Total	Range
Gyne T	Cavity	130	8.7	20.9	1127	1–36
	Isthmic	16	8.1	8.2	130	1–24
	Missing	2	2	—	4	2
Multiload	Cavity	142	5.4	5.1	761	1–24
	Isthmic	13	7.5	6.4	97	1–24
	Missing	2	15.5	—	31	1–30
Nova T	Cavity	83	3.0	4.6	247	1–24
	Isthmic	5	3.0	3.9	15	1–10
	Missing	1	15.0	—	15	15
Gravigard 7	Cavity	46	7.9	9.8	364	1–42
	Isthmic	9	8.3	9.1	77	1–24
	Missing	1	3.0	—	3	3
Lippes Loop	Cavity	9	71.6	70.2	644	1–169
	Isthmic	1	50.0	—	—	50
Various/	Cavity	68	11.5	22.2	785	1–36
unknown	Isthmic	2	23.0	—	46	22–24

Table 9.10 Pregnancy Pearl Index, by location of IUD

Cavity $\quad \dfrac{1200 \times 6}{3937} = 1.8$

Isthmic $\quad \dfrac{1200 \times 9}{409} = 26.4$

Missing $\quad \dfrac{1200 \times 3}{53} = 67.9$

Total $\quad \dfrac{1200 \times 18}{4399} = 4.9$

Nemes, G. and Kerenyi, T. D. (1971). Ultrasonic localization of the IUCD. *Am. J. Obstet. Gynecol.*, **109**, 1219–20

Piiroinen, O (1972). Ultrasonic localization of intrauterine contraceptive devices. *Acta Obstet. Gynecol. Scand.*, **51**, 203–7

Winters, H. S. (1966). Ultrasound detection of intrauterine contraceptive devices. *Am. J. Obstet. Gynecol.*, **95**, 880–2

10
Uterine metrology in Mexican women

L. REYNOSO, G. ZAMORA, M. GONZALEZ-DIDDI, M. LOZANO and R. AZNAR

Most family planning programs offer IUDs for fertility regulation; the protection against unwanted pregnancies afforded by the IUD is well documented. The most common causes for abandoning the method are bleeding and pain (Population Report Series, 1979, 1982). While the chemical constituents, and physical properties such as size, shape and elastic memory have been extensively studied, little attention has been paid to the size of the uterine cavity of IUD users. There are a few studies looking at uterine measurements of different ethnic groups and, as a rule, one IUD size is considered suitable for all women.

This study assesses the uterine size of Mexican women relative to the size of available IUDs.

SUBJECTS AND PROCEDURES

Only clinically healthy, volunteer women attending the IMSS Family Planning Clinics were included in the study, and 584 women requesting an IUD insertion agreed to have their uterine measurements taken prior to device insertion. All measurements were taken by one person and only one type of plastic metrology device was used (Battelle uterine caliper donated by Plata of Mexico). The measurements were performed without medication.

The Battelle's metrology device is a modified plastic wing sound instruction (Figure 10.1). The device is closed by pulling ring 'O', and inserted throught the cervix as a simple probe. When the uterine fundus is reached, the depth is read off the slide (total uterine length). When the 'O' ring is released, the two arms open until resistance of the lateral wall is felt and other measurements are read on the scale. The process is performed at different depths, to produce a grid map of the uterine cavity. While the metrology device is being withdrawn, the point of maximum width is identified as well as the 'point of waisting', when cavity width suddenly narrows. Total uterine length (uterus and cervical canal), endometrial cavity length, maximum width and width at waisting are recorded (Figure 10.2). Uterine

119

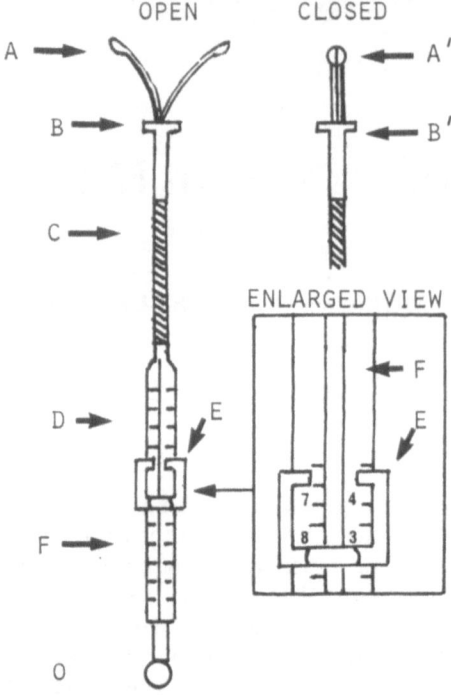

Figure 10.1 Uterine metrology device. A = wing sound open, A' = closed; B = cervical stop; C = spring to tension cervical stop; D = measuring slot; E = width measure; F = axial length (depth) slot

cavity measurements are calculated using a trapezoidal rule. The area of the cervical canal is not considered, as the cervix should not be occupied by the IUD.

RESULTS

The mean age for the group of women was 29 years, with a median within the third decade of life (Table 10.1). Mean parity was 2.7 deliveries, with a median of 2 deliveries (Table 10.2). Endometrial length and number of pregnancies are shown in Table 10.3.

A positive correlation was found between endometrial length and number of deliveries. Statistically significant differences in endometrial length were found in women with para 0 and/or 1, as compared with the rest of the group. However, maximum width did not have a correlation to the number of deliveries, although the uterine surface area increased in size with an increase in the number of deliveries. Endometrial surface area was different ($p < 0.05$) in women para 0 and 1 — as compared to the rest of the group.

Frequency distribution of uterine cavity length is presented in Table 10.4; 77.4% of the group had less than 40 mm. Tables 10.5 and 10.6 represent frequency distribution of uterine maximum width and endometrial cavity

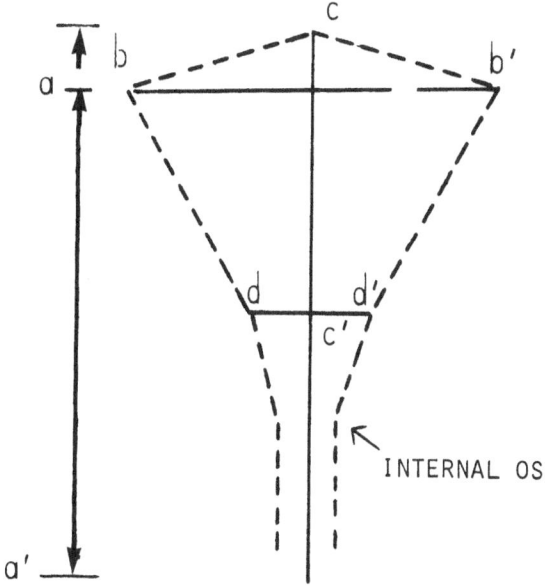

Figure 10.2 Measurements taken from uterine cavity. a − a′ = axial length; b − b′ = maximum width; c − c′ = endometrial cavity length; d − d′ = 'waisting' width

Table 10.1 Age distribution

Age distribution	Number	%
15–20	41	6.9
21–25	151	25.9
26–30	176	30.2
31–35	106	18.2
36–40	78	13.4
>40	32	5.4
Total	584	100.0

Mean $\pm$ ISD = 29 $\pm$ 6.5 years

area, respectively; 79.3% of women had a uterus of less than 30 mm maximum width and 46.3% had less than 6 cm² of uterine cavity surface area.

DISCUSSION

Measurements of uterine cavity length and uterine surface area have been previously reported using different techniques of instruments including wing sound (Hasson, 1974), the cavimeter (Kurz, 1981), planimeter hysterograms (Tejuja and Malkini, 1969), and ultrasound (Wittman and Chow, 1976). In general, these studies have reported similar results.

121

BIOMEDICAL ASPECTS OF IUDs

Table 10.2 Number of deliveries

Parity	Number	%
0	38	6.5
1	98	16.8
2	152	26.0
3	114	19.5
4	69	11.8
5	113	19.4
Total	584	100.0

Mean $\pm$ ISD $= 2.7 \pm 1.5$

Table 10.3 Uterine cavity measurement in Mexican women*

Para	0	1	2	3	4	5
Number of women	38	98	152	114	69	113
Length (mm)						
X̄	35.1†	36.8†	38.6	38.7	37.9	39.6
SD	6.4	5.8	6.4	5.9	6.4	7.1
Maximum width (mm)						
X̄	24.5	25.6	26.3	25.2	27.3	26.7
SD	6.7	5.3	5.3	5.8	6.6	5.5
Uterine area (cm²)						
X̄	5.97‡	6.53‡	6.99	6.63	7.02	7.04
SD	1.9	1.9	2.1	1.8	2.3	2.1

* Measurement taken with Battelle wing sound device; † $p < 0.01$; ‡ $p < 0.05$

Table 10.4 Frequency distribution of uterine cavity length

Length (cm)	No. of cases	%
20–30	106	18.2
31–40	346	59.2
41–50	129	22.1
51–60	3	0.5
Total	584	100.0

Hasson (1974) noticed differences between black and white groups in the US. Tejuja and Malkini (1969) in a small sample of Indian women found a positive correlation between women with small uterine cavities fitted with relatively large IUDs and the number of side-effects associated with IUD use. Our measurements of age structure and number of deliveries in a normal Mexican population compared favorably with similar data reported in the Mexican National Fertility Survey (1978).

The mean uterine length for our study group, 3.78 cm, was comparable

Table 10.5 Frequency distribution of uterine maximum width

Maximum width (mm)	No. of cases	%
15–20	71	12.2
21–30	392	67.1
31–40	114	19.5
>40	7	1.2
Total	584	100.0

Table 10.6 Frequency distribution of endometrial area

Surface (cm²)	No. of cases	%
2.0–5.0	150	25.7
5.1–8.0	328	56.2
8.1–11.0	88	15.0
11.1–14.0	18	3.1
Total	584	100.0

to others such as Hasson (1974), who reported a 3.3 cm average in the white population and a 4.2 cm for the black population and Newton (1984), who in a pilot study using the Battelle sound instrument, reported a waisting depth range from 2.7 to 3.1 cm.

The average length of IUDs presently in use varies from 3.5 to 3.8 cm; however, in our study group (Table 10.4) the frequency distribution demonstrates that 77.4% of women had an endometrial length of less than 40 mm.

Hasson et al. (1976) recommend the use of an IUD when the uterine cavity length is larger than the IUD length, by no more than 2 cm; our data indicate that IUDs may be longer than the uterine cavity in more than 50% of our population. The average maximum width in our group was 2.59 cm. This value is smaller than that reported by Newton (1984) (3.1–3.5 cm), but in agreement with Kurz's data. Kurz (1981) suggests that the transverse dimension of an IUD need not be longer than 28 mm. In our sample, 79.3% of women had uterine maximum widths of less than 30 mm.

In our study the average uterine cavity surface area was 6.69 cm² and almost half of the sample had a uterine surface area of lessk than 6 cm². These values are smaller than these reported by Newton (1984) (7.5–9.5 cm²). The area occupied by the Lippes Loop D is around 9 cm²; this IUD appears to be too large for our population. Expulsions and discontinuations for bleeding and pain noted with this IUD could be due to a size discrepancy between uterus and the device. In fact, most commercially available IUDs appear to be larger than would be comfortable for the majority of Mexican women. Smaller IUDs are needed for our population, to increase continuation rates by decreasing expulsion, pain and bleeding: the major causes for discontinuation of IUD use.

References

Hasson, H.M. (1974). Differential uterine measurements recorded *in vivo*. *Obstet. Gynecol.*, **433**, 400–12

Hasson, H.M., Berger, G.S. and Edelman, D.A. (1976). Factors affecting intrauterine contraceptive device performance. I. Endometrial cavity length. *Am. J. Obstet Gynecol.*, **126**, 973–81

Kurz, K.H. (1981) Avoidance of the dimensional incompatibility as the meain reason for side effects in intrauterine contraception. *Contracept. Deliv. Syst.*, **2**, 21–9

Mexican National Fertility Survey (1978). Encuesta Nacional de Prevalencia en el uso de metodos anticonceptivos. Julio-PPctubre, Mexico

Newton, J. (1984) Pilot study using the Battelle uterine metrology device, to measure the uterine cavity, in non-pregnant patients. Unpublished data

Population Report Series B, 64 Number 3, May (1979)

Population Report Series B. 116 Number 4, July (1982)

Tejuja, S. and Malkini, P. (1969). Clinical significance of correlation between size of uterine cavity and IUCD, a study of planimeter-hysterogram technique. *Am. J. Obstet. Gynecol.*, **105**, 620–7

Wittman, B.K. and Chow, T.S. (1976). Diagnostic ultrasound in the management of patients using intrauterine contraceptive devices. *Br. J. Obstet. Gynaecol.*, **83**, 802–8

11
Mathematical models of IUD – uterine relations

H. DERSHIN and H. M. HASSON

It has been clearly established that uterine size and shape vary considerably among different individuals. In order to fit intrauterine devices (IUDs) to the size of the endometrial cavity, Hasson (1971) developed a metrology device capable of differentiating total uterine length into cervical and endometrial components, *in vivo*. This device, Wing Sound I, is a probe with wings that expand to a diameter of 12 mm. Using the sound as a probe, with the wings folded, permits measurement of total uterine length; withdrawing the device, with the wings extended, serves to identify the uterine area which is 12 mm in width. This uterine width level defines the lower boundary of the endometrial cavity. It should be noted that the 12 mm uterine width level is an arbitrary line that does not necessarily identify the position of the anatomic internal os. This end-point is useful, however, in differentiating total uterine length into cervical and endometrial components and in defining the endometrial cavity in geometric terms.

We have studied fresh hysterectomy specimens and observed that the uterus may be described in terms of three distinct geometric zones: a lower canal-like structure with an essentially constant normal cross-section, the cervical canal; a transitional zone, the isthmus; and an upper segment with the transverse cross-sectional configuration of an isosceles trapezoid, the endometrial cavity (Hasson and Dershin, 1981) (Figure 11.1). The cavity can be modelled geometrically, with the top of the fundus representing the superior boundary of the trapezoid, the lateral uterine walls the sides of the trapezoid and the arbitrary, but fixed, dimension of 12 mm, serving as the inferior boundary. The uterine isosceles trapezoid is shown in Figure 11.2 with various segments of the trapezoid defined symbolically in Figure 11.3. In this figure (d_0) is the arbitrary 12 mm dimension representing the lower boundary of the endometrial cavity, (d_1) is an intermediate cavity width, seprated from (d_0) by a distance (l_1), (d_2) is the fundal transverse dimension; (L) is the effective endometrial cavity length and (β) is the uterine fundal base angle.

The geometry of the trapezoid requires that the segments be related to each other in terms of the following equations:

$$d_2 = d_0 + (d_1 - d_0)(L/l_1)$$

$$\beta = \tan^{-1} \left(\frac{2l_1}{d_1 - d_0} \right)$$

In order to obtain such data it is necessary to identify not only the uterine parameters attained with Wing Sound I: d_0 (the 12 mm uterine width level serving as the lower boundary of the endometrial trapezoid) and L (endo-

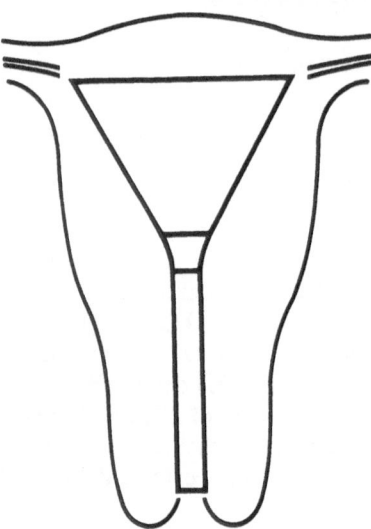

Figure 11.1 Geometric model identifying the endometrial, isthmic and cervical segments of the uterus

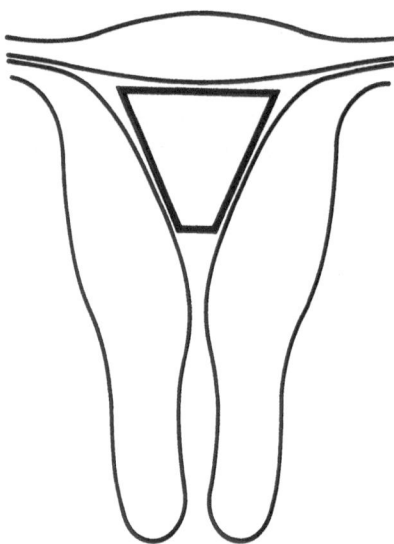

Figure 11.2 Graphic representation of the uterine isosceles trapezoid

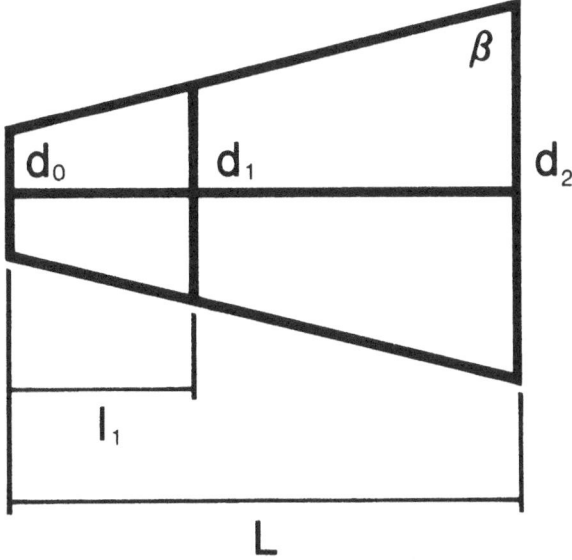

Figure 11.3   Geometric parameters of the uterine isosceles trapezoid

metrial cavity length) but also d_1 (an intermediate cavity width of predetermined dimension) and l_1 (the distance between d_1 and d_0). To accomplish this goal, the Wing Sound I was modified so as to provide not one but two stable wing spreads (of 12 and 18 mm). By using Wing Sound II as a probe, with its wings folded, one can measure total uterine length, then by withdrawing the sound with its wings extended to 18 and 12 mm, respectively, one can establish the insertion depth at which the width of the uterine cavity matches each of the predetermined wing spreads and thus gather all the information needed to identify the geometry of the endometrial trapezoid (Hassan and Dershin, 1981).

In previous experiments, good correlation was noted between fundal transverse dimensions and uterine base angles obtained by direct measurements and by mathematical computation as well as between data derived from the use of Wing Sound II and those obtained by direct measurements. Correlation coefficients of 0.85 and 0.96 were obtained for d_2 and angle β respectively, at the 99% confidence level (Hasson and Dershin, 1981).

PARAMETRIC REPRESENTATION

Given that the endometrial cavity can be ideally modelled as an isosceles trapezoid, the next step is to create a framework that will collectively capture the significant dimensions of the endometrial cavity as well as those of the IUD. This may be accomplished by displaying the defining equation parametrically, and placing the inferior boundary of the cavity (d_0) at a fixed width dimension of 12 mm. The significance of the parametric graph is that each point in the two-dimensional space represents a single combi-

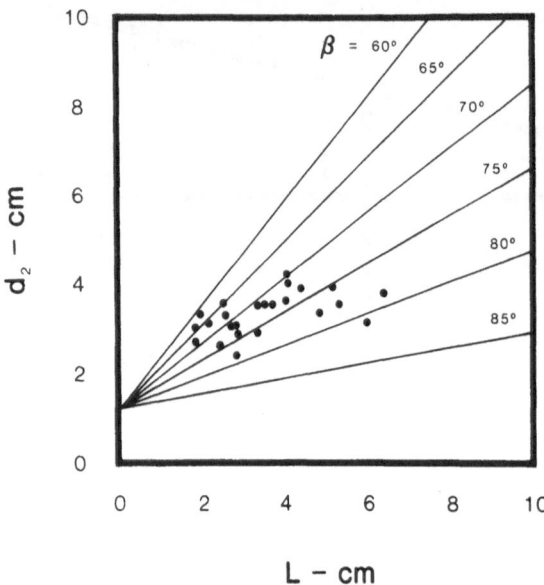

Figure 11.4 Theoretical relationships between endometrial cavity dimensions displayed in a parametrical graph. Each dot represents the axial and transverse dimensions of an endometrial cavity, obtained from fresh hysterectomy specimens

nation of uterine cavity dimensions. Conversely, every endometrial cavity can be represented by a point on the graph.

To illustrate the use of the parametric graph, all of the endometrial dimensions collected in our previous laboratory study are displayed in Figure 11.4. It can be seen that the data have a fair amount of scatter in terms of the parameters (L) and (d_2). In fact, a correlation coefficient developed solely in terms of these two parameters is only 0.56. However, the data clearly seem to fall into a pattern, with effective cavity length (L) varying between 2 and 6 cm, transverse fundal dimensions (d_2) between 2.5 and 4 cm, and fundal base angles (β) between 65° and 80°. The small size of the sample, and the *in vitro* nature of the method does not allow one to make any conclusions. However, the clustering does suggest a possible area of research that could be pursued further. While Figure 11.4 displays quite graphically the wide variability in endometrial cavity dimensions, it also suggests that it might be possible to define a boundary zone (or zones) within which one could describe, at various levels of statistical confidence, most cavities. Such zones may be found to be age-, race- or parity-dependent.

WINDOW-OF-BEST-FIT CONCEPT

It was previously shown by Hasson *et al.* (1976) that IUD performance could be correlated with cavity length. High event rates were obtained when the length of the IUD equalled or exceeded the length of the endometrial cavity or when it was shorter by 2 cm or more. It was suggested that devices occupying the lower segment and isthmus can be expected to be associated with high expulsion and medical removal rates, and possible pregnancy if the upper segment is not covered by the IUD. Devices that protrude into the cervical canal are also more prone to expulsion (Hasson, 1980).

An enhanced understanding of these phenomena, in two dimensions, can be obtained using the parametric relationships shown in Figure 11.4. Since each point in the space of the graph represents a combination of dimensions and hence a single endometrial cavity, it is possible to geometrically relate a particular IUD to all possible cavity configurations. For example, it is possible to define the combination of uterine dimensions in which an intrauterine device just touches the cavity walls and does not extend into the cervical canal. Stated differently, placement of an IUD with known length and width dimensions into the parametrical uterine graph can be shown by a specific line that distinguishes the combination of uterine dimensions into which the IUD would fit perfectly. For any IUD, such a line may be referred to as the line-of-best-fit. In Figure 11.5, the parametric graph of cavity dimensions is partitioned by the line-of-best-fit for the Lippes Loop.

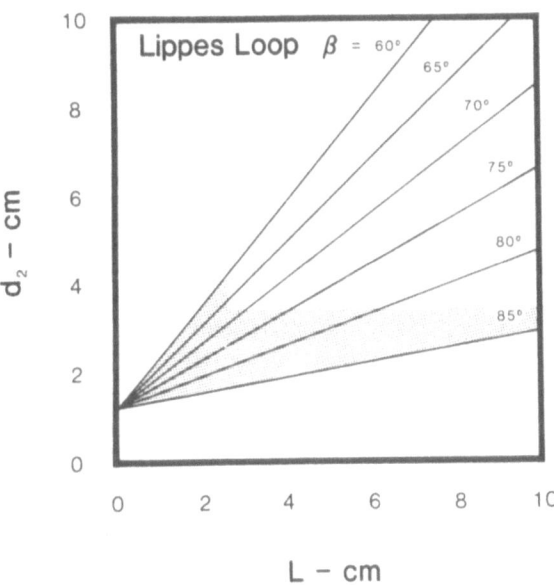

Figure 11.5   Line-of-best-fit for the Lippes Loop IUD

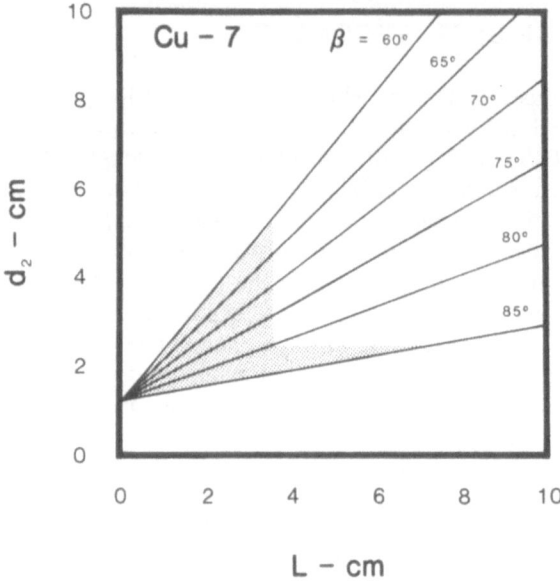

Figure 11.6   Line-of-best-fit for the Cu-7 IUD

In this diagram, the shaded zone represents all endometrial cavities that will cause Loop compression or may force the Loop to extend into the cervical canal. The unshaded zone represents endometrial cavities in which the Loop would fit loosely. Similar diagrams can be constructed for any IUD. Those relating to the CU-7 and CU-T (the Tatum T) IUDs are shown in Figures 11.6 and 11.7.

It would not be realistic to expect that the line-of-best-fit would have clinical significance since it would be unreasonable to require an IUD to fit the cavity perfectly in order for the device to perform optimally: minor geometric disproportions between IUD and static cavity dimensions are not likely to be associated with clinical events. However, it may be possible to identify degrees of IUD/uterine disproportions that do achieve clinical significance and to find that for each IUD there exists a specific zone or 'window' of uterine dimensions, overlapping the line-of-best-fit, within which the IUD does perform optimally. Such a 'window' is shown conceptually in Figure 11.8. Below and to the left of this window, one might observe events related to device compression. Above and to the right of the window, one might again find increased event rates. It is possible that the relative size of the window as well as its location on the graph would vary for different IUDs depending on their geometric and mechanical properties. IUDs that are well designed and constructed may have a larger window than those that are not.

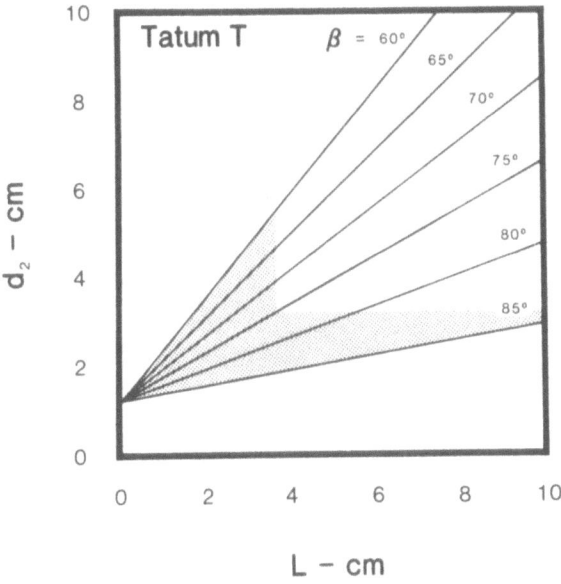

Figure 11.7   Line-of-best-fit for the Tatum T IUD

WING SOUND II NUMAGRAD AND UTERINE GEOMETRY PLOT

The process of determining d_2 and β can be simplified, and the calculation step eliminated, through use of a nomograph. Figure 11.9 demonstrates a nomograph developed for a Wing Sound II instrument with wing spreads of $d_0 = 12$ mm and $d_1 = 20$ mm, using conventional methods. Although the current Wing Sound II device has wing spreads of 12 and 18 mm, this older model can be employed for demonstration. To use the system, one enters the values of L and l_1 as measured by Wing Sound II on the nomograph. Connecting the two points with a straight line determines the transverse fundal dimension d_2. The fundal base angle β is also determined from the measurement of l_1. The usefulness of the nomograph is enhanced by the uterine geometry plot, Figure 11.9. This graph is drawn to a centimeter scale allowing the clinician to transfer the measured dimensions to a graphical layout. The ordinate of the plot is the effective endometrial cavity length L and the abscissa is one-half the transverse fundal dimension, $d_2/2$. Thus, Wing Sound II measurements of the uterine cavity can be visually displayed on the uterine geometry plot. To obtain a visual sense of the fit of any particular IUD, one merely places the actual device on the scale drawing of the cavity cross-section, as demonstrated in Figure 11.10.

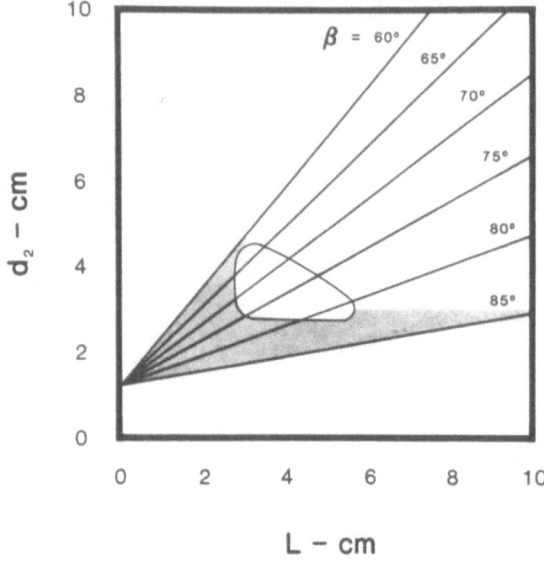

Figure 11.8 Theoretical concept of a window-of-optimum-fit for a given IUD

CONCLUSIONS

Previous work relating IUD performance to endometrial cavity length has been extended to consider the width and angularity of the cavity as well as the two-dimensional nature of the device. New instruments and methods have been devised and are being tested. Further research in the area of IUD fitting will probably lead to a better understanding of IUD performance as well as an improved and more appropriate use of such devices.

ACKNOWLEDGEMENT

This work has been supported in part by a grant from the Program of Applied Research on Fertility Regulation, Northwestern University under AID Contract AID/DSPE-C-0035.

MATHEMATICAL MODEL OF IUD – UTERINE RELATIONS

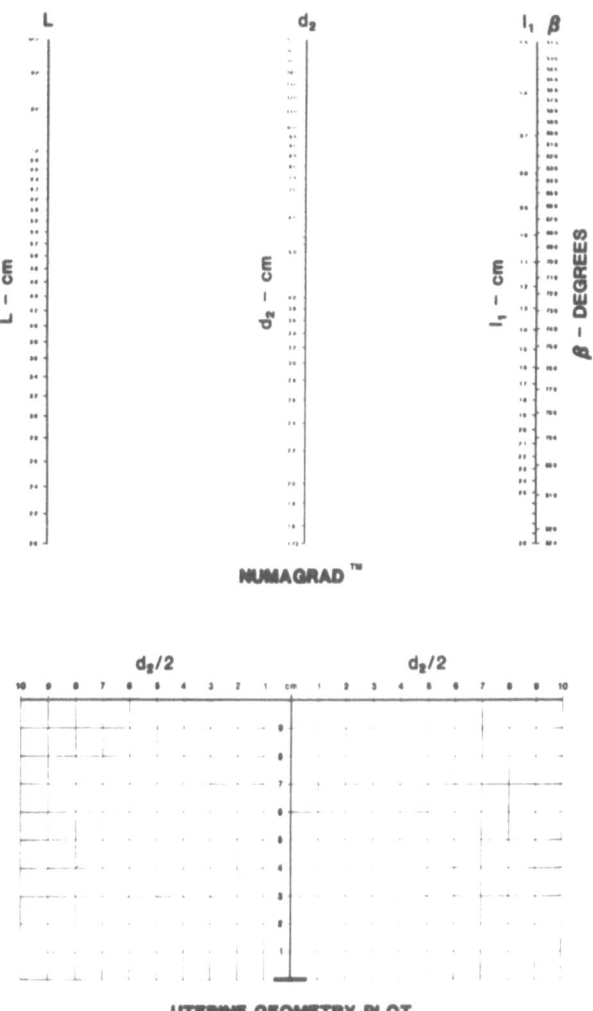

Figure 11.9 Wing sound II Numagrad and uterine geometry plot

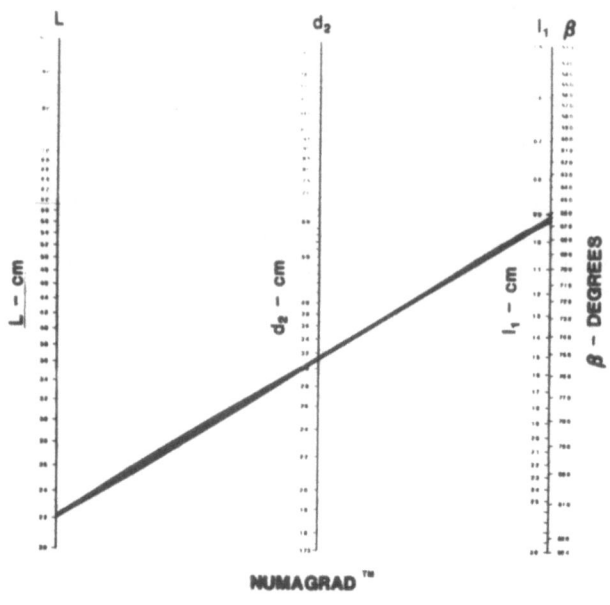

NUMAGRAD ™

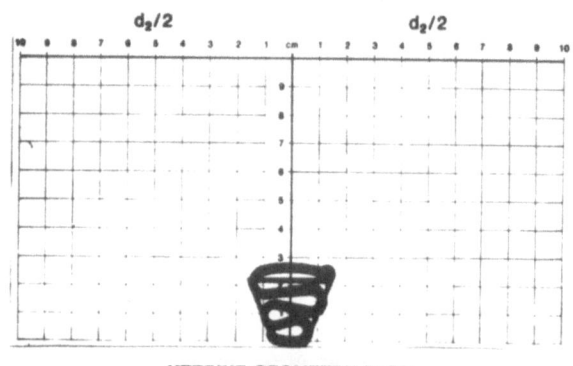

UTERINE GEOMETRY PLOT

Figure 11.10a

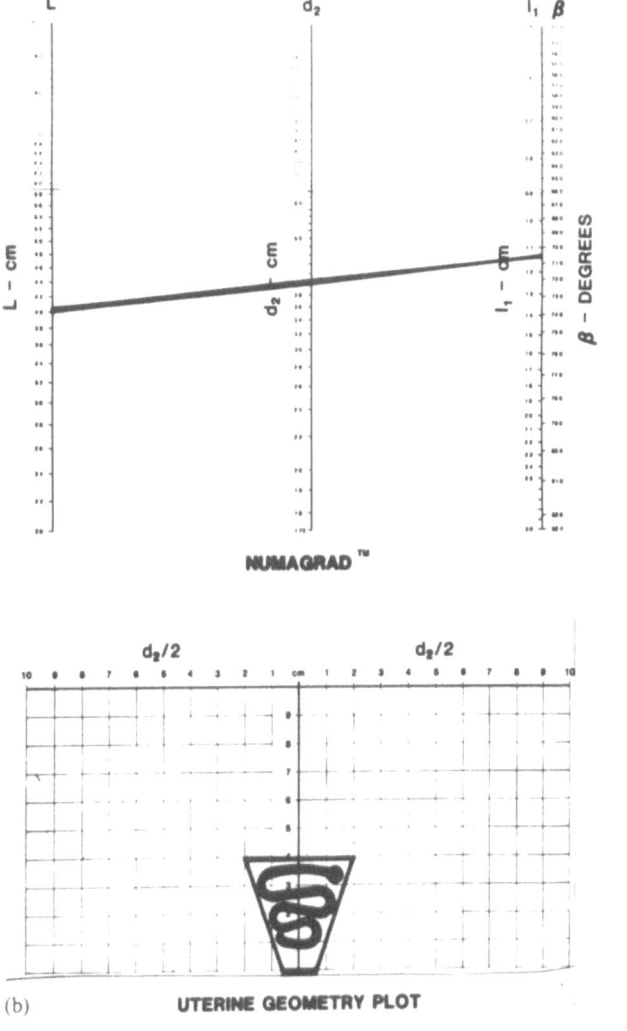

Figure 11.10 Application of the Numagrad and uterine geometry plot demonstrating (a) appropriate and (b) inappropriate fit with the Lippes Loop IUD

References

Hasson, H. M. (1971). The Wing Sound: a new uterine measuring device. *Obstet. Gynecol.*, **35**, 915-8

Hasson, H. M. (1980). Uterine geometry and IUD performance. In Hafez, E. S. E. and van Os, W. A. A. (eds.) *Medicated IUDs, Physiological and Clinical Aspects*. pp. 11-21. (The Hague: Martinus Nijhoff)

Hasson, H. M., Berger, G. S. and Edelman, D. A. (1976). Factors affecting IUD performance. I. Endometrial cavity length. *Am. J. Obstet. Gynecol.*, **126**, 973-81

Hasson, H. M. and Dershin, H. (1981). Assessment of uterine shape by geometric means. *Contracept. Deliv. Syst.*, **2**, 59-75

Index

contraceptive
carcinogenic risk with 31-3
and menstrual hygiene 33, 34
and microbial flora of cervix 33 4, 35,
36
and cervix, carcinoma-inducing
effects 26, 27, 31 2
and endometrium, morphological
effects 29
progestogen as 51 2
and sexual activity, frequency
correlation 36 7
copper IUD
contraceptive action 3
and cervix, carcinoma 31 7
and coitus, frequency 36 7
and endometrium, morphological
effects 29 30
and pelvic inflammatory disease 71, 78
and transtubal sperm migration, effects
of 37 9
and uterine wall, perforation by 79
see also named types
copper 7 IUD
insertion, discomfort during, with topical
uterine anaesthesia 92 3
line-of-best-fit for 130
and pelvic inflammatory disease 71, 78
ultrasonography of 99, 101, 110, 111
copper T IUD
and abortion 82
line-of-best-fit for 130, 131
ultrasonography of 99, 100, 110, 111
corpus luteum, and IUD-induced
prostaglandin release, in animals 46
curcumin, and IUD-induced uterine
inflammation 48
cyproterone acetate, and cervical mucus 53

Dalkon shield
insertion, discomfort during 95
and septic abortion 82
decidua formation, and progesterone-
releasing IUD 5-21
decidual cell
and Arias-Stella reaction 18 19
characteristics of 9, 11-12, 13, 19
formation, ultrastructure, and
progesterone-releasing IUD 7-12
with long term use of 14 17
glycogen content, and progesterone-
releasing IUD 6
decidual granule, ultrastructure, and
decidual response, progesterone-
releasing IUD 9, 10, 11, 12, 14 15,
20
decidual response, ultrastructure, under
progesterone-releasing IUD 5-21

and Arias-Stella reaction 18-19
electron microscopy of 7-12
K-cell 12-14
light microscopy of 5-6
with long term use of 14-17
dexamethasone, and IUD-induced uterine
inflammation 48
dictyosome, ultrastructure, and decidual
response, under progesterone-
releasing IUD 7, 8
Döderlein bacilli flora, and cervix,
carcinoma 33, 34, 35, 36

ectopic pregnancy
and Arias-Stella reaction 21
and IUD use 80-1
management 81
and pelvic inflammatory disease 80-1
emetine, and intracervical device 55
endometrial cavity
as isosceles trapezoid 125-7
parametric representation 127-8
size, and IUD, window-of-best-fit
concept 129-31
endometrial granulocyte *see* K-cell
endometrial stroma
cell morphology, and menstrual cycle 4
decidual response, ultrastructure, under
progesterone-releasing IUD 4-21
and Arias-Stella reaction 18-19
electron microscopy 7-12
K-cells 12-13
light microscopy 5-6
with long term use of 14-17
endometrium
adenocarcinoma, and copper IUD 31
and copper IUD, morphological
effects 29-30
detection at cervix 30-1
decidual response, ultrastructure, under
progesterone-releasing IUD 4-21;
see also endometrial stroma
foreign body reaction, and IUD 25-6
copper IUD 29-30
hyperplasia, and intracervical device,
animal studies 54
and IUD,
effects on 3
relationships, mathematical models
for 125-33
IUD-induced inflammatory changes, in
animal models 45-8
and anti-fibrinolytic drugs 48
and anti-inflammatory drugs 47-8
cellular inflammation 45-6, 48
edema 46
enzyme release 47
fibrinolysis 47, 48

INDEX

mechanical injury 45, 48
plasminogen activators 47
prostaglandin release 46, 48
vascular changes 46, 47, 48
leukocytosis 25-6
measurements
and IUD size, correlation 123
methods 119, 120
variation 120, 123
see also endometrial cavity
stroma cell, morphology *see* endometrial
stroma
endoplasmic reticulum
rough, ultrastructure, under progesterone-
releasing IUD 7, 8, 11
smooth, formation, and Arias-Stella
reaction 18-19
epinephrine, and topical uterine anaesthesia,
for IUD insertion 96
epsilonaminocaproic acid, and IUD-induced
fibrinolysis 48
estrogen, as contraceptive, side efects 51

fibrin, and decidual response, under
progesterone-releasing IUD 15
fibrinoid, and decidual response, under
progesterone-releasing IUD 15, 17,
20
fibrinolysin, and IUD-induced inflammation,
in animals 47, 48
fibrinolysis, and decidual response, under
progesterone-releasing IUD 47, 48
foreign body reaction, of endometrium
and IUD contraceptive action 3, 25-6
copper IUD 29-30, 38-9
fungus, and pelvic inflammatory disease, in
IUD users 74, 78

golgi apparatus, ultrastructure, and decidual
response, under progesterone-
releasing IUD 7, 8, 9-10, 11
golgi vesicle, ultrastructure, and decidual
response, under progesterone-
releasing IUD 7, 8, 9
glycogen
and decidual response, under
progesterone-releasing IUD 7, 8, 9
and K-cell 13, 14
of K-cell 5, 13, 14

Haemophilus (*gardnerella*) *vaginalis*, and
cervix, carcinoma 34, 35
heparin, and IUD-induced inflammation, in
animals 46-7, 48
Herpes simplex virus
and cervical intraepithelial neoplasia 27,
32-3
and cervix, carcinoma 33

histamine, and IUD-induced inflammation,
in animals 46-7, 48
hypertension, and progestogen 51
hypothalamic-pituitary function, and
progestogens, effect on 53
hysterectomy, and intracervical device,
studies 569

ibuprofen, and IUD-induced fibrinolysis 48
indomethacin, and IUD-induced
fibrinolysis 48
uterine inflammation 48
inert IUD
contraceptive action 3
uterine wall, perforation by 79
intracervical device 51, 52
benefits of 53-4
and cervix, effects on
bacteriological 57-9
histological 57, 58
development
animal studies 54-5
clinical trials 55-7
hysterectomy study 56-9
progestogen delivery by 51-2, 53-4
IUD
and abortion 81-2
displacement, and pregnancy,
ultrasonography to prevent 109-16
expulsion, confirmation of 79
and ultrasonography 106, 107
fitting correctly, and
ultrasonography 99-107
and foreign body reaction 25-6
length, average 123
line-of-best-fit 129-31
location
and pregnancy, occurrence 115-16
and ultrasonography 109-16
lost
complications arising from 78-80
ultrasonographic investigation 106,
107
and menometrorrhagia 77
mode of action 25-6
and pelvic inflammatory disease, risk
factors for 65-74
IUD-related 66-7, 78
micro-organisms, prevalence 72-4, 78
user-related 66-7, 78
and pregnancy
ectopic 80-1
intrauterine 81-2
prevention by ultrasonographic
testing 109-16
ultrasonographic study of 105, 106
and progestogens, local delivery of 53
side effects 3

139

INDEX